THE EXERCISE COACH®

THE EXERCISE COACH®
NUTRITION PLAYBOOK™

Gerianne Cygan, Certified Health Coach and Co-Founder of The Exercise Coach®

The information provided in this book is designed to provide helpful information on the subjects discussed. This book is not meant to be used, nor should it be used, to diagnose or treat any medical condition. For diagnosis or treatment of any medical problem, consult your own physician. The publisher and author are not responsible for any specific health or allergy needs that may require medical supervision and are not liable for any damages or negative consequences from any treatment, action, application or preparation, to any person reading or following the information in this book. References are provided for informational purposes only and do not constitute endorsement of any websites or other sources. Readers should be aware that the websites listed in this book might change.

ISBN: 1537156101
ISBN 13: 9781537156101
Library of Congress Control Number: 2016913698
CreateSpace Independent Publishing Platform
North Charleston, South Carolina

Nutrition and wellness is a complicated topic. There are as many approaches as there are experts. Yet, for an individual, nutrition and wellness is more than just a topic. It's a crucial endeavor. It's literally at the heart of one's vitality and legacy. This makes direction invaluable.

I have watched my wife Gerianne take many challenges in life head-on. In fact, it's sort of her specialty. If you have a problem, Gerianne knows there is a solution out there to be found. More than a decade ago, this led her to a journey of deep exploration and personal nutrition experimentation. After years of health issues, Gerianne committed to "fixing" her body through whole-food nutrition. As a result of this transformation, her passion led her to study Health Coaching, and she began to bring resources and education to bear on our fitness brand The Exercise Coach®.

In the last several years, as a result of her influence and efforts, our brand has helped our clients across the country live healthier lives and lose thousands of pounds.

Now, Gerianne has painstakingly undertaken the challenge of gathering into one resource the most vital information for personal health transformation, created first for our beloved clients but also for anyone interested in feeling better, looking younger, and making the most of the life God has given them. The Exercise Coach® Nutrition Playbook™ takes the complexity out of healthy eating, and at the same time gives readers an opportunity to gain a deeper understanding of how whole-food nutrition and whole-effort exercise work to optimize health, fitness, and functionality.

The Exercise Coach® Nutrition Playbook™ is not intended to be the last word on every debatable issue. In fact, it is a humble and balanced approach that allows the reader to learn, make choices, draw their own conclusions, and apply what they are ready for.

I wholeheartedly recommend the playbook to anyone looking to take his or her life to the next level through healthy eating and exercise. It is required reading for every one of our hundreds of certified exercise coaches around the country, and our go-to educational resource for the clients we care for.

Brian Cygan
Co-Founder & CEO of The Exercise Coach®
Proud husband of the author

TheExerciseCoach.

Playbook Contents

Forward · v

Introduction · xi

Welcome · xiii

Gaining an Understanding ·xvii

The Three Troublemakers · 1

Troublemaker #1 – Systemic or "Silent" Inflammation · · · · · · · · · · · · · 1

Troublemaker #2 – High Blood Sugar · 3

Troublemaker #3 – Poor Digestive Health · 4

The Super Villains · 6

Super Villain #1 – Sugar · 6

Super Villain #2 – Grains and Starchy Foods · · · · · · · · · · · · · · · · · · 9

Super Villain #3 – Dairy Products · 10

Super Villain #4 – Legumes and Soy · 12

Super Villain #5 – Artificial Sweeteners, additives like MSG, and thickeners like Carrageenan · · · 15

Super Villain #6 – Processed/Prepackaged Meals · · · · · · · · · · · · · · · 17

Super Villain #7 – Alcoholic Beverages · 17

What Should We Eat? · 19

Good-source Protein · 19

Vegetarian Protein · 19

Supplemental Protein · 20

Vegetables · 21

Fruits · 22

Healthy, Good Fats · 23

Herbs, Spices, Seasonings, and Condiments · · · · · · · · · · · · · · · · · · 24

Beverages · 25

Summing up your meals · 27

Portion Sizes · 27

Organic Foods – why they are the better choice · · · · · · · · · · · · · · · · · · 30

Glycemic Load vs. Glycemic Index · 32

Let's Talk Nutrients · 34

    Fatty Acids / Fats · 34

    Omega-6 vs. Omega-3 Fatty Acids · 35

    Antioxidants · 36

Digestive Health · 37

    Microbiota and Probiotics · 37

    Fiber · 38

Food Allergies, Intolerance, and Sensitivities · 40

Genetically Modified Organisms (GMO's) · 42

Seafood: How to pick your seafood wisely · 43

The Exercise Coach® Supplement Guide · 44

The 30-Day Metabolic Comeback Challenge™ · 46

    The Challenge is ON! What Foods are Eliminated? · 46

    What will I eat for 30 days? · 47

    Preparing for The 30-Day Challenge · 50

    Expectations · 52

    Post 30-Day Challenge · 54

Life After The 30-Day Metabolic Comeback™ · 56

    80/20 Health for a Lifetime Plan™ · 56

    Eat Daily · 56

    Eat Often · 57

    Eat Sometimes · 57

    Eat Rarely · 57

    Never Eat · 58

The journey to a less toxic existence · 59

The Exercise Coach® RESOURCE AND REFERENCE Guide · · · · · · · · · · · · · · · · · · 61

    Sample menu for The 30-Day Metabolic Comeback Challenge™ · · · · · · · · · · · 61

    Recipes · 73

    Vegetarian Addendum · 75

    Meal Planning for the 30 Day Metabolic Comeback™ · · · · · · · · · · · · · · · · · · · 77

    Food Journal · 79

    Testimonials · 81

    After the 30-Day Metabolic Comeback™ Food Reintroduction Journal · · · · · · · · · · · · 83

    Fat Loss: Fact vs. Fiction · 84

    Healthy Oils · 98

    Healthy Snack Ideas · 100

Resource and Reference Links · 103

Alcoholic Beverages · 103

Artificial Sweeteners · 103

Bone Broth · 103

Books On Nutrition, Healthy Living · 103

Butter · 104

Cancer · 104

Carrageenan · 104

Cholesterol: Debunking the Myths · 104

Coconut Water · 105

Dairy · 105

Diabetes, Insulin Resistance, High Blood Sugar · · · · · · · · · · · · · · 105

Eggs · 105

Environmental Toxicity · 105

Fats · 106

Fiber · 106

Fish Oil · 106

Fodmaps · 106

Food Sensitivities, Allergies · 106

GMOs (Genetically Modified Organisms) · · · · · · · · · · · · · · · · · · · 107

Grains · 107

Glycemic Index (GI) And Load (GL) · 107

Gluten · 107

GMO Foods · 107

Inflammation · 107

Legumes (beans / soy / peanuts) · 108

Meats · 108

Msg And Other Additives · 108

Natural Health Care, Beauty, And Personal Hygiene Products · · · · 108

Non-Toxic Cleaning And Laundry · 109

Nuts · 109

Oils · 109

Organic Eating · 110

Organic, Pure Spices · 110

Plastic · 110

Probiotics · 110

Seafood Buying And Information · 111

Shopping: Sources For On-Line, Healthy And Organic Food Products· · · · · · · · · · · · · · · · · ·111

Soy ·111

Sugar ·111

Vitamins And Nutrients · 112

Water · 112

Websites On Nutrition, Healthy Living, Recipes· 112

Introduction

I'm excited that you are taking a step toward better overall nutrition and health, and continuing in your quest for further knowledge and understanding. My hope is that you will be inspired to begin your whole-food eating journey, or continue to improve the path you may already be on. Ultimately, my goal is for you to achieve outstanding metabolic indicators for your health, at any age: healthy weight, blood pressure, cholesterol and blood sugar levels; and optimally functioning cells, digestion, and brain.

When most people think about nutrition, the word diet automatically comes to mind, also weight loss and fat loss. I can assure you, if you follow the general guidelines laid out in this play-book regarding exercise, and primarily eat the healthy, whole food choices that you will find in our lists Eat Daily and Eat Often, you will lose weight (assuming you are not over-eating even healthy foods). You will look and feel much better, at a healthy weight. But, what is even more important is that the weight loss, along with the proper exercise and healthy nutrition, will also be a factor in the improvement of the other metabolic indicators I mention above. And this means you have a better chance of feeling more energetic, enjoying more activity, looking younger, and living longer! Aren't those the things we all desire?

Thank you for taking the time to read The Exercise Coach® Nutrition Playbook™. I truly hope it will inspire you to make whatever change you need, at whatever stage you are at in life and health.

Gerianne Cygan, Certified Health Coach and Co-Founder of The Exercise Coach®.

Welcome

Welcome to The Exercise Coach® Nutrition Playbook™. We believe nutrition goes hand in hand with our exceptional exercise program, and together give you the keys to great health, weight management, longevity, and exceptional daily living.

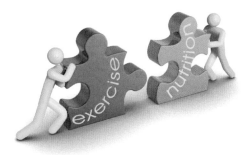

A whole range of biochemical processes occur in our bodies on a daily basis. This is known as metabolic function. At The Exercise Coach®, we help people achieve optimal metabolic function with the perfect combination of whole-effort exercise and whole-food nutrition. It's our secret weapon called: The Metabolic Comeback™.

The Exercise Coach® Metabolic Comeback™ program is unique! Nowhere in the country does technology merge with accountability like they do at The Exercise Coach®. The combination of these two key ingredients, plus our private studio setting, gives you a *one-of-a-kind* client experience that delivers the results people truly want.

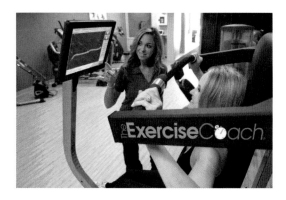

The Metabolic Comeback™ is not a 7-day, 30-day, or any set-number-of-days, program. It's The Exercise Coach's® ongoing combination of whole-effort exercise and whole-food nutrition. Within the Metabolic Comeback™ we offer shorter, 30-day periods, which we call The 30-Day Metabolic Comeback Challenge™. This is a time of metabolic reset, a time to gain greater understanding of your personal eating habits, and a time to learn what foods may or may not be causing you issues such as allergies, sensitivities, weight gain, skin rashes, fatigue, etc. More information on The 30-Day Metabolic Comeback Challenge™ is found later in this guide.

So what exactly do we mean by whole-effort exercise? To put it simply, The Exercise Coach® uses modern, smart-technology to generate a customized strength goal based on each person's ability to generate force throughout a set range of motion. Then, we ask you, the client, to generate enough effort, or as we like to say – "give it your **whole** effort" -- throughout the entire set to reach the customized goal our highly-trained and certified exercise coaches set for you, individually.

Did we tell you that it only takes 20 minutes? One of the most challenging concepts for those new to The Exercise Coach® to believe is that our workouts only last about 20 minutes. The reality is that the benefits of exercise are NOT realized by moving around or engaging in random activity for long periods of time, but by forcing the body, and specifically our muscles, to activate and contract to the greatest degree possible in a short period of time. Whole-Effort is the secret ingredient that forces a cascade of wonderful benefits that improve every system of our body.

The Exercise Coach® has systemized and harnessed the most effective and safest way to ask your body, in all its uniqueness, to generate the necessary effort to cause change to occur: Right Intensity Training™. Right Intensity Training™ is based on the user's ability, history, and current joint-muscle function, and is designed to foster precisely the appropriate effort to unleash maximal adaptation.

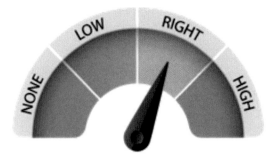

What's really exciting is that every system of our body can achieve a positive adaptation. This includes our muscular system, circulatory system, skeletal system, neurological system, digestive system, respiratory system and endocrine system. Our clients also see improvements such as increased muscular strength, lower blood pressure, reduction or reversal of type II diabetes, improved heart health, stronger bones, improved brain function, the reduction of cellular inflammation, and a slowdown of the aging process.

The second component of The Exercise Coach® Metabolic Comeback™ is whole-food nutrition --the focus of this Playbook. What exactly is whole-food nutrition? Put very simply, a whole food is a one-ingredient food product that does not need any processing to make it edible, like meat, fish, eggs, vegetables, fruits, legumes, nuts and seeds. In practice this means we eat meals that contain whole ingredients, as well as healthy oils, fats, herbs and spices, plenty of pure water, and low or no sugar or starch. And when it comes to whole-food choices, those that are nutrient-dense (meaning packed with nutrients) are your very best choices.

At The Exercise Coach®, we hope that once you experience the way you look and feel doing The Metabolic Comeback,™ you will never want to turn back!

Gaining an Understanding

We are all biochemically unique. What works for one may not necessarily work for another. The purpose of The Exercise Coach® Nutrition Playbook™ is to guide you toward eating whole, nutrient- dense foods that will prove beneficial for your individual body. One person may do very well, for example, choosing broccoli as his go-to veggie, while someone else may experience intestinal discomfort every time he eats it! Remember, even the healthiest food can prove to be damaging to someone allergic or sensitive to it. Of course, there are fundamentals to great, whole-food eating which benefit everyone. We hope to guide you through those fundamentals to help you learn which foods are the most beneficial for your body, so you can avoid troublemakers (see below), and lead a healthy, energetic, and long life.

If you wish to discover a more in-depth, scientific understanding of any of the concepts mentioned here, peruse the reading list in our Resource and Reference Links, page 103. The Exercise Coach® Nutrition Playbook™ is not intended to rewrite what is already written very well and readily available. It is intended to be a clear, concise guidebook on *why* you need to eat whole foods (*to avoid the troublemakers*), *which* whole foods you should eat, and *which* foods you should avoid or limit. *What* you eat is then up to you! We hope that after giving whole-food eating a go, you enjoy a new lifestyle of eating fresh, whole foods, and discover that they taste even better than processed, sugary foods that rob you of your good health.

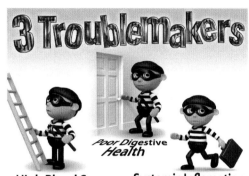

The Metabolic Comeback™ (Whole-Effort Exercise + Whole-Food Nutrition) focuses specifically and looks to conquer three troublemakers wreaking havoc in your body – systemic inflammation, high blood sugar, and poor digestive health. Both components of The Metabolic Comeback™ address these troublemakers in different ways, and together, help you build up an amazing defense against what these troublemakers cause – a whole host of diseases and accelerated aging. This playbook will focus specifically on the nutrition side of The Metabolic Comeback™; the exercise side will be addressed with your Certified Exercise Coach during your scheduled workout sessions.

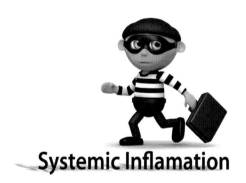

TROUBLEMAKER #1 – SYSTEMIC OR "SILENT" INFLAMMATION

The first troublemaker is Systemic Inflammation. Inflammation is an unhealthy condition for your body, yet one many people are suffering from, sometimes silently! When we think of inflammation, we typically think about a sprained ankle, a bump on our head, or other physical markers pointing out injury. In these cases, inflammation is our body's signal that we are injured and we need healing. That's a good thing! We then typically do something to allow our bodies to heal (ice compress, rest, therapy, anti-inflammatory medication or supplements). This type of inflammation is what is commonly referred to as classical or acute inflammation. But this is NOT the silent, systemic, cellular inflammation we are talking about here.

Systemic/silent inflammation at the cellular level is the single greatest cause of health problems today. Over 70% of our country's health care costs stem from silent inflammation, because it leads to a long list of diseases including heart disease, diabetes, cancer, dementia, migraines, autoimmune diseases, digestive diseases, and accelerated aging. It often exists without having "pain" as a symptom. But after years and years of continued inflammatory attack, chronic disease and organ damage can set in. This is a very serious condition, and can be quite complicated to understand. It is only through proper diet, adequate nutrients, rest, and stress reduction - which includes The Exercise Coach® Metabolic Comeback™ - that we can reduce this type of inflammation. Unfortunately, there is no magic pill! (Please read The Exercise Coach® Blog Post by T.J. Lux, dated April 24, 2014) http://blog.exercisecoach.com/muscle-quality-and-inflammation/.

The Exercise Coach® Nutrition Playbook™ centers around anti-inflammatory food choices - foods that will not add to silent inflammation, and foods that can combat existing cellular inflammation. Remember, some healthy, whole foods may not be problematic to some, but may be inflammatory to others due to allergies or sensitivities. But then there are foods that quite simply, are inflammatory to just about everyone. We will discuss those individually in later sections of this guide.

The ideal way to find out if you have silent or systemic inflammation is through blood testing. Your doctor will be able to order some of these tests for you, including high sensitivity C-reactive protein testing. Depending on your symptoms and initial blood test results, your physician may order more specific testing. Some symptoms that can indicate the presence of systemic inflammation are: (1) craving carbohydrates; (2) ongoing fatigue; (3) being overweight; (4) waking up groggy; (5) brittle fingernails; (6) unhealthy cholesterol profile, and; (7) high blood pressure.

Acute or classic inflammation typically goes away in a short period of time. But we can suffer from chronic systemic inflammation for years! Our cells, tissues, and organs can remain in an inflammatory state that may eventually lead to weight gain and disease.

Here are the major contributors that can lead to chronic inflammation: toxic and unhealthy diets, insufficient omega-3 intake, excessive omega-6 intake, stress, lack of sleep, environmental toxins, poor oral health, smoking, excessive alcohol use, lack of exercise, over-training with your exercise regimen, and poor gut health (Troublemaker #3).

By following The Exercise Coach® Nutrition Playbook™, we believe you will greatly reduce inflammation in your body. Combined with our safe and effective exercise program, you will see changes in short periods of time that will continue as long as you are committed to the overall program.

In addition, numerous studies and our experience have shown that taking pharmaceutical-grade fish oil may dramatically improve your inflammatory profile. Some supplements such as Vitamin D3 and curcumin have also been touted as having a powerful anti-inflammatory effect throughout the body. (See The Exercise Coach® Supplement Guide later in this playbook).

Americans are the fattest people on the planet and suffer the most inflammation. Yet, it is possible to turn things around in your body through diet and exercise, even in as little as 30 days!

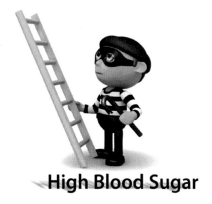

High Blood Sugar

TROUBLEMAKER #2 – HIGH BLOOD SUGAR

According to The American Diabetes Association, 86 million people have pre-diabetes (about 27% of the population!). And, these people are five to six times more likely to eventually battle Type II Diabetes (known also as adult onset) over time. What is pre-diabetes? It is a condition when people have consistently high blood glucose (blood sugar) levels that are higher than normal, but not reaching the point of full-blown Type II Diabetes. Full-blown Diabetes affects approx. 29.1 million people (9.3% of the population) and is a condition where your body produces too little insulin or uses it ineffectively. *

Pre-diabetes and Type II Diabetes are sadly common, yet largely preventable. Full-blown type II Diabetes is a problem where blood glucose levels rise to much higher-than-normal levels, and stay elevated longer than they should. At that point, your body is not using insulin (your blood sugar reducing hormone) properly. This is called insulin resistance. Insulin is a necessary storage hormone. In a healthy body, insulin efficiently unlocks muscle and liver cells for the body's glucose (sugar) to be stored away as glycogen (stored carbohydrate used for energy) for the body to use at a later time.

Deconditioned muscles and poor nutrition are root causes of insulin resistance. Weak muscles are less responsive to insulin's actions. In other words, weak muscles don't listen to insulin's commands, and they don't reduce and store the blood sugar like they need to. In that distress, the body produces **really high** amounts of insulin to force that glycogen (or blood sugar) out of the bloodstream. Chronically poor nutrition also creates insulin resistance by consistently exposing your body to elevated sugar and insulin levels. The result is the same as it is for weak and deconditioned muscles: a dangerous lack of responsiveness to insulin -- a panic situation for your body.

So, when your body experiences insulin resistance, there is one place for the sugar to end up. It's converted to triglycerides (which are an unhealthy blood fat) and the door is then wide open for storage of triglycerides in our fat cells. Chronically high insulin and continual fluctuations in blood sugar result in fat storage and cellular distress.

Simply put, bad carbohydrates (sugars, starches, and processed foods) start the whole process in the first place by increasing blood sugar… and high blood sugar is toxic!

The Exercise Coach® Nutrition Playbook™ is focused on encouraging you to eat whole foods that won't increase your blood sugar to high levels, and in fact, have been shown to reduce your existing high blood sugar to a much lower or even normal level.

People who have Type I Diabetes do not produce their own insulin and therefore, take insulin injections to regulate their blood sugar. This condition is not caused by nutrition and cannot be prevented the way Type II or Adult Onset Diabetes can be prevented and even reversed. Type II diabetes is what is being discussed under the "High Blood Sugar" discussion.

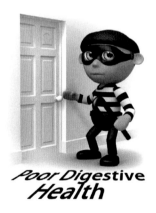

Poor Digestive Health

TROUBLEMAKER #3 – POOR DIGESTIVE HEALTH

The last big troublemaker The Metabolic Comeback™ can help improve is Digestive distress. Because of poor eating habits over many years, people suffer greatly from a variety of conditions that originate in the digestive tract. This can include heartburn, reflux, ulcers, constipation, diarrhea, gas, bloating, and a variety of other intestinal and/or bowel disorders. Worse, as time goes on, many people develop what is known as "leaky gut" syndrome where food particles are being released into the blood stream due to holes in the intestinal walls. This is toxic, and for some, results in an autoimmune response from our bodies. Our bodies are literally fighting off these invaders!

Leaky gut and poor digestive health can manifest in many ways such as autoimmune diseases, celiac disease (severe gluten allergy), other food allergies, intolerances or sensitivities, eczema or other skin conditions, general allergies, and asthma, just to name a few! In other cases, the immune system simply becomes weaker and weaker, causing increased susceptibility to sickness like colds, flu, fatigue, headaches…and the list goes on).

Your digestive system needs good bacteria (microflora). Everyone has good and bad microflora in his or her intestines. A balanced and well-functioning digestive system is critical for your overall health – from your brain to your organs, to your entire immune system. * Since 65% of your immune system is in your intestinal lining, you can see why protecting it is so important.

A diet of poor-choice carbohydrates (sugar, starch, processed foods) will help the bad microflora flourish and crowd out the good bacteria that keeps your intestinal mucosal lining intact. If you are someone who has extreme digestive issues, you need to follow a diet that eliminates all poor-choice carbohydrates, until you are healed. The Exercise Coach® Nutrition Playbook™ focuses on whole foods that are healing, not harmful, to your gut.

As you can see, all three major troublemakers have the same solution – reducing or eliminating sugars, starches, and processed/fake foods. And, a healthy body is achieved in the same way – through whole-foods that do not include an over-abundance of sugar, starches, or processed/fake foods.

*"The interconnectedness of your gut, brain, immune, and hormonal system is impossible to unwind. The past few years have brought a scientific flurry of information about how crucial your microflora are to your genetic expression, immune system, body weight, and composition, mental health, memory, and minimizing your risk for numerous diseases." – Dr. Joseph Mercola, Mercola.com.

The Metabolic Comeback™ (whole-effort exercise + whole food-nutrition) is an excellent way to reduce or eliminate the troublemakers from your life – permanently! The exercise portion contributes greatly, even by itself. Combined, the combination sets you up for even greater success.

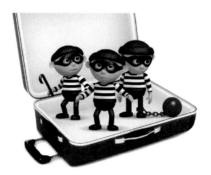

Send those troublemakers packing

There are certain foods that are largely responsible for the three troublemakers (inflammation, high blood sugar, and poor digestive health) gaining access into your life to begin with. These foods are what we call the **Super Villains**, and we recommend you avoid or reduce them as much as possible: sugar and other sweeteners, highly processed grains, gluten, and starches, most dairy products, soy and some legumes, processed/pre-packaged meals; and alcoholic beverages.

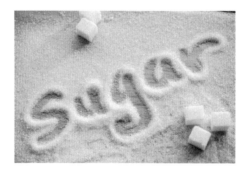

SUPER VILLAIN #1 – SUGAR

It's probably safe to assume that this is not a moment of enlightenment for you to hear this. Today, everyone knows, or has heard, that sugar is not good for you. For those who already suffer from any of the three troublemakers, eliminating sugar is the best solution. (There, we said it!). In even 30 days of avoiding sugar, you will probably feel a big difference and be on your way toward healing.

Sugar is a carbohydrate, including refined and natural, white granulated sugar (table), brown sugar, sanding sugars, powdered sugar, coconut sugar, malt syrup, molasses, agave nectar, honey, maple syrup, cane juice cane sugar, corn syrup, high fructose corn syrup, fructose, date sugar, coconut sugar, palm sugar, malt sugar, rice syrup, sugar cane, and turbinado (raw).

As you can see, the list is quite extensive, and on an ongoing whole-food lifestyle, it is recommended that you reduce or avoid foods that contain any of these sugars.

If you want to lose weight, if you want to reduce inflammation, if you want to avoid diabetes, if you want to have a balanced digestive system – you have to avoid sugar.

Q&A
Why not natural sugars? Don't they contain nutrients?

The answer is yes; some natural sugars do contain great nutrients. That is why fruit is a whole food that we recommend on The Metabolic Comeback™ (except for those who are trying to heal from one of the three Troublemakers). Raw, local honey has some nutritional value. When you are on the 80/20 *Health for a Lifetime Plan* (see page 56) you may use it.

What about "natural" sweeteners like stevia, xylitol, erythritol, monk fruit sweetener, or other sugar alcohols from plants? Can I use those?

In small quantities, some of the naturally occurring, plant-based sweeteners listed above are accepted on the Metabolic Comeback™ over the other sweetener choices. While there is always controversy surrounding lesser-known choices, these sweeteners have been used for centuries in other cultures without any evidence of harm. If you do choose to use xylitol, erythritol or other sugar alcohols, it is best to go easy because too much, to quickly, can cause gas or diarrhea in some people. And, it is important to make sure these sweeteners are a pure form, and not a special processed form (like the brand Truvia®, for example, which is chemically modified Stevia). Most of these sweeteners are found in health food stores or are an ingredient inside of some healthy-alternative protein bars or shakes. Some typical snack or beverage products are also starting to include them.

Fruits contain fructose and other sugars. Why is it ok to eat them?

Fructose outside of the fruit is one of the worst sugars you can eat. Research shows that fructose is a major contributor to insulin resistance, and significantly raises triglycerides, which can lead to heart disease. Fructose is also a direct cause of belly and love handle fat, which is associated with a greater risk for diabetes, heart disease, metabolic syndrome, and even fatty liver disease. Outside of fruit, avoid fructose, high-fructose corn syrup, and agave nectar.

Within the fruit there are much lower concentrations of sugars, including fructose. The glycemic load is far reduced when eating the whole, nutrient-dense fruit, than eating only its juice, or eating fructose as a sweetener. Whole fruit contains lots of fiber, which slows down the absorption of the sugar in the blood stream. And, some fruits (like raspberries or strawberries) contain much less sugar than others (like ripe banana or papaya). For those who are trying to lose weight or have type II diabetes or metabolic syndrome, we recommend a smaller daily consumption of fruit or possibly none for a period of time. For others, adjust to your body's individual needs but by all means, eat fruit! (See Glycemic Load, page 32).

What about fruit juices?

Fruit juices do contain nutrients but as we discussed above, they are missing the fiber. Drinking a glass of fruit juice is simply drinking a glass of sugar that will spike your blood sugar levels immediately. Better to choose the whole fruit, or use your Vitamix or other powerful blender to blend the fruit into a smoothie type drink where the fiber remains. Veggie Smoothies with protein powder and fruit added is a great choice!

Sugars, in summary

In terms of our 3 Troublemakers: (1) Sugar triggers the release of inflammatory messengers called cytokines. * (2) Sugar raises blood sugar, which can lead to insulin resistance, which can lead to Type II Diabetes and obesity; and (3) Sugar feeds the bad bacteria in your digestive system and allows it to flourish. If that's not enough, sugar is the chosen "food" of cancer and according to multiple studies, can lead to cancer. Sugar also increases your risk for heart disease, leads to obesity, harms your teeth, disrupts your hormones, and is addictive!

Keep in mind – every person's biology is unique. Generally speaking, people who are already healthy and active (exercise regularly, especially strength training and those on The Metabolic Comeback™) may tolerate more sugar than people who are inactive, overweight, and eat a Western, high-carb, high-calorie diet. And that's why we advocate balance and ultimately desire everyone to be on the 80/20 Health for a Lifetime Plan. (See page 56).

*American Journal of Clinical Nutrition

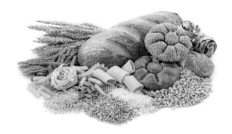

SUPER VILLAIN #2 – GRAINS AND STARCHY FOODS

A grain is the seed of a plant that is used for food. Primarily, a grain product is any food made or processed from wheat, rice, oats, corn, barley, millet, and so on. Starchy foods to avoid are generally anything made from grains (bread, pasta, chips, crackers, cereals, etc.) as well as white potatoes and white rice. Grain and starch products are carbohydrate-dense and nutrient-poor (meaning, you are basically eating sugar, without gaining a great deal of nutrition). As such, they promote chronically elevated insulin levels that can lead to systemic inflammation and all the diseases that may result. Grains also contain some inflammatory components that can cause damage to your intestinal lining and can ultimately lead to what we were speaking of in Troublemaker #3 – Leaky Gut Syndrome.

There are a *few* whole grains that are nutrient-dense and can be a part of a regular diet if eaten just a few times a week by those who are healthy. These are steel-cut oats; quinoa; brown rice and buckwheat. You can make the dish even more nutritious and have less affect on blood sugar by combining these grains with a healthy fat and protein source. Remember, we are speaking of eating the grain, not flour made from the grain. And, if you have systemic inflammation, diabetes, cancer, or are highly affected by blood-sugar spikes, even these grains are not for you!

Q&A
But aren't whole grains better for you?

The question is, better than what? Perhaps in the lineup of better to worse, and assuming you are going to eat grains as a part of your diet, whole grains certainly are a better choice (if they truly are WHOLE grains, minimally processed). Remember, all flours, even those made from whole grains, are refined and highly processed carbohydrates. While they may contain minimal nutritional value over white flour, the effects on your blood sugar levels, your metabolism, and your hormones are the same! Your blood sugar will spike! All in all, they are not the top choice for people who want to eat foods that keep inflammation down, keep blood sugar and insulin well- regulated, and keep digestive health at its best.

Aren't gluten-free flours healthy for you?

For those with celiac disease (an allergy to the protein gluten) gluten-free flours are the only flours they can eat without getting very ill! But many people, knowingly or unknowingly, are also "sensitive" to gluten (meaning the gluten proteins cause bad reactions such as bloating, gas, headaches, joint pain, brain fog, fatigue, skin rashes, etc.).   Therefore, gluten free flour is a better choice for them as well. However, while gluten-free flours may alleviate some of the symptoms caused by gluten-containing flours to those allergic or sensitive, they still have the same effects on the human digestive tract as any other processed flour or starch we discussed above. For that reason, all flours and simple starches should be considered a sugar and should be avoided.

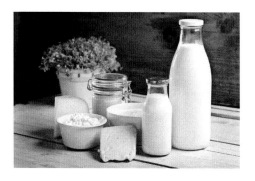

SUPER VILLAIN #3 – DAIRY PRODUCTS

Dairy is any food product made from the milk of an animal. Of course, if we really think about it, milk is for babies' nutrition and therefore, cow milk is for baby cows, goat milk is for baby goats, and so on. We can argue that dairy is full of nutrients, but many would also argue that the nutrients are designed for consumption by those of the same species. Not to mention: in any given species, mother's milk is meant for the intensive growth spurt experienced by its babies, not adults! Food for thought!

Although dairy has been consumed and tolerated for years, specifically by people of European, Middle Eastern, and Indian descent, the purpose of good nutrition is not to find foods our bodies will simply tolerate but to find foods that will actually promote great health. And this is where dairy falls short. The carbohydrate portion of milk, the lactose, together with the milk protein, namely casein, produce a surprisingly high insulin response, which we now know is inflammatory to our body and promotes disorders like obesity and diabetes.

Also, non-organic dairy products contain hormones and antibiotics because the dairy cows they come from are treated with those substances. Those cows eat an unnatural diet of grains which is harmful to their digestive system and are saturated with pesticides – so, this type of milk does NOT DO OUR BODIES GOOD.

Dairy is high on the list of food allergens and on the list of foods that harm the gut lining (can cause leaky gut). And, dairy is often a food group that many people are sensitive too. Once eliminated from the diet, asthma symptoms, seasonal allergies, acne, eczema, post-nasal drip, rheumatoid arthritis, and digestive disturbances often abate significantly or even subside entirely.

For these reasons, we say avoid dairy (with the exception of organic butter or ghee) in your everyday meal planning.

If you suffer from allergies, stuffy nose, runny eyes, asthma symptoms, acne, eczema, joint pain, you just may be allergic or sensitive to dairy.

Q&A
If I tolerate dairy well, can I have it more often?

Dairy consumption is an area of controversy, and many in the nutrition world are debating its merits. While we generally do not recommend it, we leave those decisions up to you, knowing we have armed you with plenty of good information! Remember, the sugars in dairy cause a high insulin spike and this is inflammatory. In addition, dairy growth factors like IGF-1 promote unregulated cell growth — the underlying cause of cancer (uncontrolled reproduction of mutated cells). And, the proteins in dairy, especially casein, are also inflammatory, and have been associated with increased risk of autoimmune diseases such as rheumatoid arthritis.

The milk you buy from the local supermarket nowadays has been pasteurized, ultra-pasteurized, or homogenized. The liquid is a chemically altered substance, heated to remove pathogens and bacteria and to prolong its shelf life. The resultant low-enzyme activity makes it difficult to digest as we have discussed, the altered fat content renders the vitamins and minerals difficult to absorb, and the residual drugs and antibiotics pose a threat to human health. On top of this, the naturally occurring beneficial bacteria have been destroyed. These are all reasons that continue to support reducing or eliminating typical dairy from your daily diet.

Milk from commercially raised cows is actually dangerous to consume unless it is pasteurized. Factory-farmed animals are routinely fed an unnatural, high-protein soy- and corn-based diet and given shots of BGH (bovine growth hormone) to artificially increase milk production. This diet is so contrary to their biology that it causes severe illnesses that can only be combated by continually injecting the cows with antibiotics.

If you do choose to consume dairy, even occasionally, we recommend you choose only organic products, grass-fed when possible, to eliminate added hormones, antibiotics, and pesticides. And then, choose the full-fat versions because the fat is the healthy part!

I've heard about raw milk being healthy for you. Is that true?

Today, raw milk refers to unprocessed, untreated milk straight from the cow. There are many proponents of drinking raw milk. Raw milk is an incredibly complex whole food, complete with digestive enzymes and its own antiviral, antibacterial, and anti-parasitic mechanisms conveniently built into a neat package. It is full of both fat- and water-soluble vitamins, a wide range of minerals and trace elements, all eight essential amino acids, more than 60 enzymes, and CLA—an omega-6 fatty acid with impressive effects on everything from insulin resistance to cancer to cardiovascular disease. Humankind has safely consumed raw milk in its natural state for thousands of years.

Raw milk from healthy, grass-fed, and pasture-raised cows is in a league of its own. Organically raised cows are happy, fed on their natural diet of grass and other cow-friendly foods. They enjoy access to sunshine and pasture grazing in summer, and in winter they feast on nutritious hay or silage. While that sounds nice and like a solution to eating dairy, the issue becomes availability. Many states have outlawed raw milk, and those that allow for it have many regulations. You need to check your own state and local regulations and then find local farms you absolutely trust!

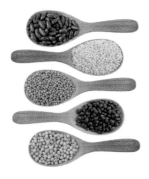

SUPER VILLAIN #4 – LEGUMES AND SOY

Legumes (other than soy)

Legumes are anything in a pod such as beans, peas, lentils, or peanuts. Soy refers to soybeans (a legume) or any food product made from soy.

While beans are a great source of fiber (see <u>Fiber</u> section, page 38), protein and minerals, for many people beans cause uncomfortable digestive issues such as gas, bloating, and diarrhea. This is why all legumes (except green beans and peas) are eliminated for our 30-Day Metabolic Comeback Challenge™. However, beans are an extremely nutrient-dense, high-fiber carbohydrate choice and can be eaten several times a week if you are not affected in this way.

One reason some diets eliminate legumes is because they contain lectins, a type of protein that can bind to cell membranes. Studies have shown that lectins can damage the lining of the small intestine, as well as harm other functions of the body. However, it is important to note that cooking neutralizes the lectins found in most legumes; 15 minutes of properly cooked legumes show low or no residual lectin activity. Finally, it is important to note that lectins are found in 53 fruits, vegetables, spices, and other commonly eaten plants – including healthy ones we recommend!

Another reason some diets eliminate legumes is because they contain phytic acid (phytate). Phytate is the storage form of phosphorus, which humans cannot digest. It binds to certain minerals we need in our bodies, and thus, prevents absorption. In addition, phytic acid interferes with various enzymes we need for good digestion. Remember: although in large amounts phytic acid is destructive, in small quantities, it is tolerable and our gut enzymes actually break down the foods that contain phytic acid to extract the nutrients our bodies need. (Spinach and Swiss chard contain five times the amount of phytates as most legumes).

Ultimately, moderate amounts of legumes, soaked and prepared properly, within the context of a diet that is nutrient-dense overall, are not harmful, and can even be helpful. But remember, many people are just plain unable to absorb the carbohydrates in legumes because eating them results in uncomfortable digestive symptoms. And, since eating legumes is not at all necessary for great health, you may just choose to skip them.

Q&A
Are peanuts good for you? They are legumes, right?

One legume that is still controversial in terms of health benefits vs. health problems is peanut and peanut oil. In light of this conflicting data, and because of other risks associated with peanut consumption, we recommend either minimizing your intake of peanuts or avoiding them entirely.

Soy – the good, the bad, and the ugly.

Soy is being separated out from all other legumes because it is one of the most controversial foods in the world! Some experts call it a superfood; others, a toxic, hormone disrupting poison! The Exercise Coach® Playbook™ is in no way an exhaustive research book on soy. Yet, we have come to the conclusion that with this much controversy, the ugly outweighs the good, and we should include it in our foods to avoid. We have shared some articles in our Resource and Reference Guide for your own study. As always, you are the ultimate judge.

Soybeans originated in the East but are now grown worldwide and on a large scale in the United States. In all forms, soybeans must be cooked since raw soy is poisonous. Soybeans are used to make many foods including tofu and soy milk, can be eaten whole in the form of edamame, and are used in fermented foods like miso, natto, and tempeh. In addition, because soy is extremely inexpensive, it is used to make soybean meal to feed livestock, soy protein, used in many processed foods, and as soybean oil, again used in lots of processed foods and deep fryers all across America. Soy is even included in many baby formulas.

THE GOOD: Soybeans do contain healthy nutrients, including manganese, selenium, copper, potassium, phosphorus, magnesium, iron, calcium, vitamin B6, folate, riboflavin (B2), thiamin (B1) and vitamin K. They also contain fiber, fat and protein. Soy has been linked to reducing total cholesterol, the risk of heart disease, and the risk of prostate cancer in mature men. (*Some studies support all of these claims; others do not*). Most people agree however, that if you are going to consume soy, you should consume in its whole (but not raw) or fermented forms (i.e., not in any of its processed forms).

THE BAD: Like all legumes, soy contains phytates and lectins and all of their unhealthy characteristics. While soybeans are a complete protein source, the amino acids are in a much weaker concentration to the protein supplied from meats or eggs. (Complete proteins are those that contain all essential amino acids in sufficient quantity). Two essential amino acids in soy protein, methionine and lysine, are present only in small amounts. This limitation means that soy protein does not compare as favorably with animal protein for some people as for others, particularly for those who have soy allergies and difficulty digesting soy protein. And, when you cook soybeans at a high temperature, the protein actually becomes denatured, and the quality reduces even further. As for the fats, they are not good fats. They are Omega-6 fatty acids, which lead to inflammation (exactly what we hope to avoid).

As well, soy contains isoflavones (active compounds) that are classified as *endocrine disrupters* – chemicals that interfere with the normal function of hormones in your body. These are known as phytoestrogens because they mimic the hormone estrogen (the female sex hormone produced in women and to a degree in men). Why is this bad? It's bad because our bodies need hormonal balance to be well. Phytoestrogens confuse our bodies and create imbalances by either stimulating our estrogen receptors, or by blocking them. In either case, our body responds poorly. For women, this can result in longer and more painful menstrual periods (or sometimes on the positive side it means a reversal of pain and heavy blood flow – but at what cost?). And, many studies have linked isoflavones to breast cancers and increased risk of breast cancers. (There are also studies showing a protective nature in some breast cancers). For men, soy has been shown to decrease sperm count, as well as have a negative effect on sexual development due to the increase of estrogen in the body.

THE UGLY: Soybeans are by far the largest GMO (Genetically Modified Organism) crop on the planet (See <u>GMO's – Frankenfoods</u>, page 42). And, unless soybeans are organic, they are sprayed heavily with Glyphosate (the chemical known as Roundup). (<u>See Organic foods, why they are the better choice</u>, page 30).

Bottom line – While the research is not cut and dried, we think you should protect your sex-hormone balance at any age. When something is this controversial, the best question you can ask is: "Does my body benefit more by eating this food, or by avoiding it?" We propose that you avoid it in all processed forms and in its oil form, and if eating in the whole or fermented forms, do so very moderately, and ONLY choose organic.

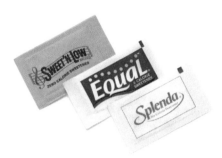

SUPER VILLAIN #5 – ARTIFICIAL SWEETENERS, ADDITIVES LIKE MSG, AND THICKENERS LIKE CARRAGEENAN

Artificial sweeteners and additives like MSG are man-made compounds or chemicals added to food products to make foods last longer and taste better, contain fewer calories, and appeal to our brain's sensitivity to sugar, causing us to crave more of those types of foods. In addition, there is plenty of research that shows toxicity to the body and the brain!

Artificial sweeteners are non-nutritive and very controversial in terms of side effects and potential health concerns. The artificial sweeteners primarily include Splenda® (sucralose); Equal®/Nutrasweet® (aspartame); and Sweet-n-Low® (saccharin). This guide will not go in-depth on the studies done on mice and the ill health affects shown. Nor, will we make a claim that a specific illness is directly caused from any of these sweeteners. There are plenty of articles and research out there already to help you get more informed (some can be found in our Resource and Reference Guide at the back of this playbook).

Studies have shown that artificial sweeteners can lead to poor digestive health and raise your blood sugar more than even regular sugars. Gut health is important to all aspects of your body's functions, including blood sugar regulation. Artificial sweeteners (all three major types) have been shown to dramatically change your gut microorganisms, particularly bad bacteria, which proliferate considerably and take over the good gut bacteria to create a major imbalance, which also leads to higher blood sugar levels. Eran Elinav, M.D., a scientist from the Weizman Institute of Science in Israel concluded, "what we are seeing in humans and also in mice is the previously unappreciated correlation between artificial sweetener use and microorganisms in the gut."

One of the most important goals throughout The Metabolic Comeback™ is freedom from the addictive properties of sugar and sweeteners. It's important to emphasize that sugar and sweeteners are highly addictive. Replacing real sugar with the artificial stuff does not break cravings or addiction to it, does not improve insulin sensitivity, and won't help you lose weight. In fact, regarding weight control, studies indicate that quite the opposite has occurred. People have become even fatter!

Artificial sweeteners do not break our cravings or addictions to sugar. They do not improve insulin sensitivity. They will not help you lose weight. In fact, studies show that people end up fatter!

Another inflammatory substance found in some food items (even those marked as healthy like some almond milk, coconut milk, nut milk ice creams and creamers) is Carrageenan. Although Carrageenan is derived from a natural source (a type of seaweed), it has been shown to be destructive in the digestive system and may lead to leaky gut and bodily inflammation. Be sure to purchase your nut milk products without this ingredient.

With regard to MSG (Monosodium Glutamate) and other similar chemical additives found in most processed foods, you should simply never eat them! MSG and other similar additives are required to be listed on all food labels. The FDA labels them as GRAS (generally recognized as safe). However, the symptoms reported due to the long-term use of these additives are: headaches, migraine, sweating, facial tightness, numbness in face and neck, heart palpitations, chest pain, nausea, and weakness. We know they are highly addictive, which means consumers want to eat processed foods containing these additives over and over again, and in large quantities. When there is a whole myriad of wonderful, healthy, spices and seasonings available, why resort to these artificial chemicals?

Finally, artificial sweeteners and chemical additives overwhelm our taste buds, making it difficult to enjoy the true flavors of real food. It's interesting how after a few weeks of eliminating these substances, clients tell us how amazingly good a particular vegetable tastes!

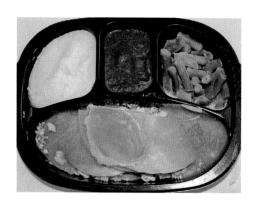

SUPER VILLAIN #6 – PROCESSED/PREPACKAGED MEALS

Processed meals are any foods typically packaged in boxes or bags for convenience. They are loaded with preservatives and other man-made chemicals and "natural" flavorings. Most Super Villains are typically ingredients in a processed meal.

While everyone enjoys convenience and saving time, we put our health at great risk for this compromise. Be very aware of packaging that says, "all natural," or "made with real....(fill in the blank)." These claims only mean something is in there that occurs naturally -- whatever that might be. And, that a smidgen of *something* "real" is also in there. *(There are plenty of "real" and "natural" things that you would not wish to be in your food).*

Often people choose processed and prepackaged meals because they claim to promote fat loss by restricting calories. But that comes with a host of other problems. If you can, choose instead to make big batches of your own whole food meals. It's better to freeze those for convenience later than to damage your body with processed foods from the freezer aisle.

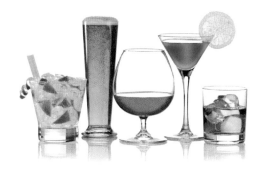

SUPER VILLAIN #7 – ALCOHOLIC BEVERAGES

We know what alcohol is, right? The drink of the gods. Think fine wines, grain alcohols like vodka, Piña Coladas on the beach! Not so fast! Alcohol is neurotoxic, which means it generally has a negative effect on your brain. It is basically condensed sugar with no nutritional value. Therefore, it does affect your blood sugar in negative ways. And, even with the health benefits described below, because many people consume large amounts and some become addicted, we do list it here as a Super Villain and not a recommended food.

Studies show that very moderate amounts of alcohol, while still having no nutritional value, may have some health benefits. "Very moderate" means up to one drink a day for an average woman, and up to two drinks a day for an average man.

Studies show that moderate consumption of alcohol offers three potential protective benefits: (1) lower risk of cardiovascular disease; (2) increased longevity; (3) assistance in prevention of the common cold; (4) lower risk of cognitive impairment; (5) reduced risk of gallstones; (6) reduced risk of Type II diabetes.

The key here is "very moderate," and also the assumption that you are currently in good health. If you are already diabetic or have cancer or heart disease, etc., we recommend that you abstain from alcoholic consumption completely. Regardless, we list alcohol on the Eat Sometimes food/ beverage list on page 57. The benefits of consumption truly only exist within this small window of opportunity; think, "less is more."

Usually, only a little more than a very moderate amount of alcohol impacts our brains and affects our decision-making. So as enjoyable as it may be, and as beneficial as red wine may be with regard to Resveratrol (a protective antioxidant), consumption of alcohol does not generally promote good health. If you currently do not drink alcohol, we do not recommend that you start simply to enjoy these potential benefits. They are present in all of the other healthy food choices listed under Eat Daily or Eat Often food lists, page 56.

S o now that we've got the super villains that do not promote good health out of the way, let's talk about the great whole foods we do promote eating at The Exercise Coach®.

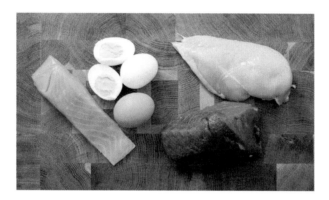

GOOD-SOURCE PROTEIN

Good-source protein is the foundation of your Metabolic Comeback™. When we say "good sources of protein" we are generally talking about proteins that come from animals found in their natural environments. While it is not a requirement that the protein you eat is organic, humanely raised, grass-fed, antibiotic- and hormone-free, or wild-caught, these are the best choices for maximum nutritional benefit and health. Eggs, meat (including beef, game, ruminants, poultry, and pork), and fish, are the preferable sources of protein at The Exercise Coach®.

If your protein sources are of the highest quality from the list above, choose cuts that include the fat. It has plenty of great nutritional value for your brain and your body. If you are going to eat traditional, store-bought meat, we advise you to choose and eat the *leanest* cuts of meat. Commercially processed meat will have traces of pesticides, antibiotics, and growth hormones residing in its fat, so you are better off eliminating it. In addition, meats that are cured or processed with sugars, sulfites or carrageenan (cured bacon, conventional sausages, jerky, lunch meats, etc.) are not considered good source protein and should be avoided.

VEGETARIAN PROTEIN

If you are a vegetarian, depending on your category/type, you may still be able to eat high-quality protein from fish or eggs. If not, then you will need supplemental protein, and protein from good plant sources like some legumes and whole grains such as quinoa or brown rice (see <u>Vegetarian Addendum</u> in the Resource and Reference Guide).

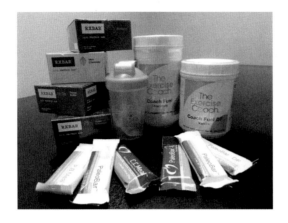

SUPPLEMENTAL PROTEIN

Protein is a very important part of a healthy Metabolic Comeback™. For some, getting enough protein through diet alone may be difficult and the convenience of high-quality protein in supplemental form is wonderful! You can easily incorporate protein powder into your veggie/fruit smoothie and sprinkle it on many of your other food dishes. The key is high-quality supplemental protein. Sadly, much of what is sold in stores (even in health food stores) is very low quality, and we would never recommend it.

Coach Fuel,™ Coach Bars,™ and RXBARS® are great sources of convenient, high-quality protein products available at The Exercise Coach®. Our Coach Fuel™ is made of the highest quality, grass-fed, non-denatured whey protein. Because of the low-heat method used, Coach Fuel™ retains the valuable enzymes pasteurization destroys. The protein maintains the full range of fragile immune-boosting components naturally present in fresh, raw milk. And finally, because of the quality of the cow the whey comes from, this small amount of good-source dairy becomes very nutrient dense. The whey protein bars are also an excellent choice, as they do not contain any artificial ingredients or non-nutritive sweeteners. Last, RXBARS® contain egg white protein and are delicious, yet simple, with less than ten ingredients.

The Coach Fuel™ Dairy Free line is a great choice for those who are sensitive or allergic to dairy, as it contains protein from non-GMO, North American yellow peas. It's a true vegan source of protein that offers excellent digestibility and nutritional benefit. There are also several different Exercise Coach® Dairy Free protein and fiber bars to choose from.

Remember, these products offer a great way to *supplement* with convenient, high-quality protein, in addition to primarily consuming choices in the good-source, whole food protein category.

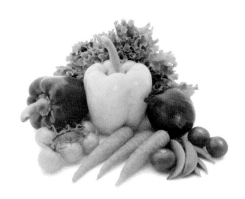

VEGETABLES

I like to call vegetables nature's primary medicine chest, because they truly help prevent disease and also help heal when disease is present. When it comes to vegetables, we recommend eating as many servings as you can with your meal, and even in between. There is truly no limit! Three, half-cup servings is the minimum, but don't stop there! Since you will be eliminating high-calorie sugars and starches, you will need some extra calories! Your body will benefit greatly if you choose from a wide variety of colors and seasonal varieties. Vegetables are nutrient-dense, meaning they are filled with plenty of vitamins, minerals, antioxidants, fiber, and other phytonutrients. Remember to include leafy greens, white veggies like onions, red veggies like beets, yellow/orange veggies like sweet potatoes and squash, and blue/purple veggies like cabbage and eggplant. We provide a full list of most veggies in the <u>What Should Be On My Plate</u> resource, page 48.

Grandma was right: Eat your Veggies! Eat as many servings as you want and be sure to eat a wide variety of types and colors.

Q&A

Are there specific ways I need to prepare/cook my veggies – or are they better for me raw?

While there are many benefits to eating raw veggies, some are even healthier when you cook them. Therefore, if you enjoy raw veggies, keep enjoying and add more choices. Vegetables may be eaten raw, steamed, boiled (but only to al dente), baked, roasted, grilled or sautéed. Any way you like is good, and variety is the spice of life!

Are there any vegetables that should be limited?

Starchy vegetables, which include sweet potatoes, beets, parsnips, pumpkin, turnips, and winter squash varieties, should be eaten in smaller portion sizes, and limited to three to four times per week. These vegetables have a higher sugar concentration, and therefore will affect blood sugar adversely if eaten in unlimited amounts daily.

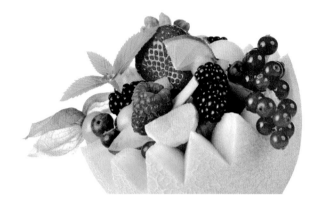

FRUITS

Fruit is full of terrific health-promoting antioxidants, vitamins, minerals and fiber. Several servings of fruit (one to three cups) each day allows you to gain the nutritional benefits from this very healthy food group. Fruit is also a "tasty" component in nature's medicine chest!

However, fruit is sweet and contains fructose (see explanation in <u>Super Villain #1-Sugars</u>), a type of sugar that generates a greater blood-sugar response than the sugars in vegetables. So if weight loss is a major goal, or if you are diabetic, we do suggest limiting yourself to two, half-cup servings per day. It's best to choose the powerhouse fruits that are lower in sugar but loaded with antioxidants such as raspberries, blueberries, strawberries and blackberries. Also, keep in mind that overconsumption of fruit may actually prevent you from breaking your brain's habit of craving sugar. If you are trying to break a sugar addiction, fruit may be a no-no until you are ready to slowly add a little bit into your diet at a later time. Last, skip fruit at breakfast. This may help you eliminate the craving for sugar throughout the day.

Q&A
Is it better to eat my servings of fruit in one sitting or spread out over the day?

Since fruit contains sugar, it is far better to eat smaller servings spread throughout the day.

What about dried fruit?

Dried fruit falls more into the category of candy than fruit. The drying process eliminates the water and condenses the sugar. For example, a half-cup serving of fresh cranberries contains two grams of sugar. A half-cup serving of dried cranberries contains a whopping 37 grams of sugar!

Most canned fruit is packed in heavy sugary syrup, which is very bad for you! Canned fruit packed in juice still contains plenty of extra sugars, and possibly more preservatives. Opt for fresh fruits whenever possible.

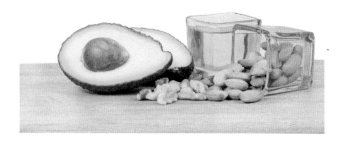

HEALTHY, GOOD FATS

Eating healthy fats is the best way to achieve optimal health and longevity, lose body fat, and maintain your healthy weight. Fat is crucial in providing you energy and ensuring you feel satisfied throughout the day, thus preventing you from feeling hungry.

Many people have lived through the non-fat, or low-fat era, the era that took out healthy fats from our diets and replaced them with unhealthy, low-fat, and fat-free foods such as processed carbohydrates, all kinds of sugars, and toxic fats such as margarines and other trans-fats; the era that made "saturated" fats a villain and created the S.A.D. (Standard American Diet) consisting of processed proteins, sugary grains and starches, plenty of other sugars, and insufficient amounts of fats (except for toxic lab-created versions). Sadly, many people still believe the lie that eating fat makes you fat, and unfortunately, they are gaining weight and becoming unhealthy as a result. Excess body fat comes from – you guessed it – sugars and starches!

The type of fat we are advocating is HEALTHY FAT. Your brain, immune system, hormones, and digestive system all rely on an appropriate amount of healthy fat. Good fat benefits you in several ways: (1) your hormones are affected positively so you have lots of energy, feel less hungry, yet burn more calories; (2) systemic inflammation is lowered (and as you know, one of our three primary goals in our whole food eating plan is low inflammation); and (3) you will feel satiated because when you eat fat, your brain sends a signal that you are full.

Healthy fat sources are primarily: animal fats, from organic, grass-fed and pastured animals; high-quality, clean-sourced fish and seafood (preferably fatty types); avocados; olives; olive oil;

raw nuts and seeds (excluding peanuts, which are a legume); organic coconut oil; organic coconut milk and other nut milks; pure nut butters; organic eggs (preferably free-range and local); MCT oil (medium-chain triglycerides); and low-sugar dark chocolate.

Bad fats (the fats that replaced our good fats in the past) are primarily trans-fats found in fast foods and packaged foods including margarines (also called hydrogenated or partially hydrogenated oils); vegetable oils, peanut oil, soybean oil, corn oil, canola oil; animal fats from factory-farmed sources; non-organic eggs; and any other fat high in Omega 6 fatty acids. (See Fatty Acids, page 35).

There are also fats that are neutral, meaning that they will add flavor but do not add any particular health benefit. Yet, they are of no detriment to your health either. You can eat them or avoid them. These include: organic palm oil; lard (from organic, grass-fed animals); and organic butter and ghee.

Remember, it's very important to make healthy good fats a part of your daily meals.

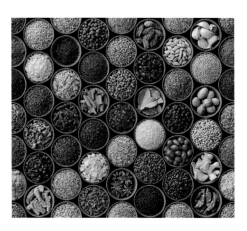

HERBS, SPICES, SEASONINGS, AND CONDIMENTS

The Exercise Coach® believes that maintaining a healthy weight does not mean you need to eat bland foods! Spice it up and you'll be amazed at how amazing fresh, whole foods can taste! If the flavor of food appeals to you, you are more likely to continue to eat that food, even if it's a healthy choice. That means weight maintenance becomes easier and you are less likely to slip back into eating poor-choice carbohydrates. Get creative. Most of these seasonings contain living plant compounds (phytochemicals) that are full of anti-aging and anti-inflammatory properties. Therefore, your already-healthy meal becomes even MORE healthy! Some of the best choices are turmeric, cinnamon, garlic, oregano, cacao, and mint. A complete list is found on our Metabolic Comeback™ What Should Be On My Plate resource, page 48).

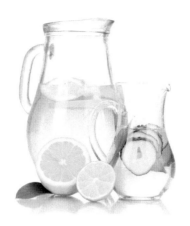

BEVERAGES

Due to the detrimental effect of artificial sweeteners, all diet sodas or other flavored beverages made with them are listed on our <u>Never Eat</u> (or drink) list.

So what should you drink? Water mostly! You may also enjoy mineral water, teas, bone broth, black coffee, and unsweetened nut milks, in addition to healthy green or Coach Fuel™ smoothies. But the importance of drinking plenty of fresh, filtered water each and every day cannot be over-emphasized, primarily to avoid dehydration (the lack of water in your body). Dehydration reduces the amount of blood in your body, making your heart pump much harder in order to deliver the oxygen you need. Also, many of your body parts (brain, blood, muscles) consist of a high percentage of water, and need to be replenished continually to function appropriately. As well…water cushions your organs, regulates body temperature, helps you breathe easier, helps convert food to energy through nutrient absorption, and removes waste! Anyone thirsty?

Q&A
What if I don't like plain water?

There are other tasty ways to enjoy fresh water: (1) add a splash of fresh lemon, lime, or mint; or (2) infuse your water with fruits or veggies (add strawberries or cucumber to your water and keep in a pitcher in the refrigerator). The water will absorb the flavor of the fruit or veggie without absorbing very much of its sugars.

How much water should I drink in a day?

Contrary to what you may hear, there is not a magic number when it comes to ounces of water everyone should drink. At the same time, two or three eight-ounce glasses probably won't cut it! Known to many is the eight, eight-ounce glasses, rule of thumb. However, bio-individuality really applies here, and you need to listen to your body. On hot days, days when you exercise heavily, or when you are sick, your body will need more water. And as you drink more water, your body craves more water!

What are the best nut milks?

Cashew, almond, and coconut are all good choices. However, it is vital that you only choose unsweetened versions and make sure that carrageenan is not included as an ingredient. (See page 15).

SUMMING UP YOUR MEALS

To sum it all up, your meal should consist of (1) a healthy protein source; (2) plenty of fresh, organic (when possible) vegetables; (3) a healthy fat source; (4) a glass of water; (5) plenty of herbs and spices to invigorate your taste buds; and sometimes (6) organic (when possible) fruit.* To help you, we have hundreds of delicious recipes on The Exercise Coach® Pinterest Page, on our Facebook Page, and on our website at www.exercisecoach.com. We also list great recipe sites in our Resource and Reference Guide, and many are included in the books we recommend. We want to make this as simple as possible!

You should plan to eat three meals per day with one to two snacks. You don't have to wake up at 6:00 a.m. to fit breakfast in, but do fit it in! A good breakfast including a great protein source, veggie, and healthy fat sets you up for an energetic morning where you don't crave sugar, and are not hungry until lunch. No time for big preparations? A delicious green smoothie made with Coach Fuel™ grass-fed whey or dairy-free protein powder, green veggies, sweeter veggies or berries, and a dollop of coconut oil will do the trick!

*Limit servings of fruit if you are diabetic or trying to lose weight. (See page 22).

PORTION SIZES

No one likes to measure or weigh the food we eat. And we don't think you should either! Instead, here are easy guidelines to help you. You may use your own hand as a guide for many foods, or remember some simple portion sizes for foods you eat regularly:

Meats and fish	One serving is about the size and thickness of your palm. Meals should include one to two palm-size portions (approximately 4-6 oz.).	
Vegetables	Both hands needed for this one! Eat as much as you can and hopefully more than one variety.	
Fruit	Close your hand to make a fist – this is about a ½ cup serving of fruit. Medium size = 1 serving (apples pears, oranges, plumbs, ½ of grapefruit). Fruit never replaces vegetables in your meals!	

Starchy veggies	Includes sweet potatoes, beets, parsnips, pumpkin, turnips, winter squash. (same as fruit, amount that fits into closed fist, about ½ cup)
Oils and butter, Nut butters	The size of your thumb is about a 1 oz. serving size. Choose one to two servings per meal.
Nuts and seeds, olives, coconut flakes	Touch your thumb to your fingers and have enough to fit inside your cupped hand. Enjoy with meals or as your snack.
Avocado	½ an avocado = one serving.
Fruits eaten	Medium size = one serving. (Apples, pears, oranges, plumbs, half a grapefruit) Whole or peeled.
Nut milks	¼ cup = one serving.
Eggs	Two per serving for the average person, three for very tall people or for those with higher protein requirements.

Relax! Exact portion size is not as important if you are primarily eating from the nutrient-dense, whole-food categories! Do your best. If you are trying to lose weight and finding it difficult, or if it just feels like too much food, cut back on your portion sizes. Not enough food? Add a little more!

Q&A
I'm having my three whole-food meals and two snacks, but I am still hungry!

Many people feel hungry when they first transition to great, whole-food eating. Most of the time it's not really hunger; it's actually a craving for poor-choice carbs or sugars. If you are really hungry, could you eat a meal of salmon and broccoli right now? Or is that not appealing? Begin to learn the difference between hunger and cravings, as well as hunger and anger, boredom, exhaustion, stress, or other emotions that make us want to eat. Emotions are powerful triggers that can lead people to eat, and many times, to overeat.

If you have determined that you ARE in fact hungry between meals, even with your snack, and not gaining unwanted weight, we recommend you increase portion sizes at mealtime. And, add a larger portion of healthy fat, along with a larger portion of protein.

My Right Intensity™ workout is performed at a very high intensity. Do I need more protein or larger snacks?

On the days that you perform your workouts, you generally need added nutrition to help you prepare for and recover from the activity. On training days, have a pre-workout mini-meal about 60 minutes prior, which will signal your body to prepare for activity. This can include a ½ portion size of protein and a healthy fat. For veggies, only include non-starchy choices. Post-workout, it's great if you are able to eat 15-30 minutes following your exercise session. This should include easily digestible protein such as egg whites, chicken or salmon; a carb-dense, starchy veggie such as sweet potato or beets; and little or no fat. Another great option pre- or post-workout is a Coach Fuel™ Smoothie, Coach Bar™ or RXBAR®. If a regularly scheduled meal falls right before or after your workout, you will not need to add any extra nutrition.

Everyone is biologically unique, and it's best to experiment with pre- and post-workout nutrition to see what benefits you the most. However, never do your workout on an empty stomach.

Organic Foods – why they are the better choice

Throughout The Exercise Coach® Nutrition Playbook™ we have recommended that you choose organic whenever possible. Sadly, eating organically grown foods is the only way to avoid the cocktail of chemical poisons present in commercially grown food. More than 600 active chemicals are registered for agricultural use in America – that's billions of pounds annually. The average application equates to about 16 pounds of chemical pesticides per person every year. The Environmental Protection Agency (EPA) approved many of these chemicals before extensive diet testing. The National Academy of Sciences reports that 90% of the chemicals applied to foods have not been tested for long-term health effects before being deemed "safe." Further, the FDA tests only 1% of foods for pesticide residue. The most dangerous and toxic pesticides require special testing methods, which are rarely if ever employed by the FDA.

We often forget that many of the pesticides we ingest come not only from fruits and veggies, but also from non-organic protein and dairy sources. Fish and animals accumulate pesticides in their fatty tissue, so when we eat the animal products, we ingest the pesticide. The animals accumulate the pesticides by eating animal by-products, fishmeal, and grains that are heavily laden with toxins and chemicals. In addition, the animals are treated with antibiotics and growth hormones that also pass into their meat and milk. (See information cited in our Resource and Reference Links, page 103).

If that wasn't bad enough, genetically engineered (GE) food and genetically modified organisms (GMO) are contaminating our food supply at an alarming rate, with repercussions beyond understanding. GMO foods do not have to be labeled in America and the lobby against this in Washington is very strong. Because organically grown food cannot be genetically modified in any way, choosing organic is the only way to be sure that foods that have been genetically engineered stay out of your diet. We understand that there are those who wholeheartedly believe that GE and GMO foods are healthy. Regardless, choosing organic is important for the other health-related reasons.

When choosing organic, be careful to read the label. 100% organic products display the USDA Organic Seal. Products marked as just "organic" are not 100% (generally 95% organic). Last, "made with organic ingredients" means simply that the product contains about 70% organic ingredients and does not bear the USDA seal.

Your budget may not allow for every produce item you purchase to be organic. The EWG (Environmental Working Group) publishes a Dirty Dozen list of fruits and veggies that test to be the most contaminated with pesticides, as well as the "Clean 15," which lists those foods that are the least contaminated. The link is provided in our Resource and Reference Links, page 110, and the list is included on our <u>What Should Be On My Plate</u> Resource, page 48.

Regarding seafood, the Monterey Bay Aquarium has a Seafood Watch program including a guide to buying the best and safest seafood (printable or via their downloadable app.; the link is included in our Resource and Reference Guide, page 111. And, the EWG also offers an abundance of information on which fish contain the highest levels of mercury and which have the lowest and highest amounts of healthy Omega-3 fatty acids.

For grass-fed, pastured meats, Eat Wild is an excellent website that will teach you about the health benefits of grass-fed meats and where to shop for them. This link is included in our Resource and Reference Guide.

Eating organic is a more expensive way to eat. However, if you eliminate or reduce buying foods like ice cream, snack chips, cookies and cakes, there should be more of your budget left over to buy organic whole foods!

Q&A
Do organic farmers also use pesticides?

According to Whole Foods, whose information is based on the latest scientific research and is updated regularly, "Organic farmers' primary strategy is prevention. By building healthy soils, healthy plants are better able to resist disease and insects. When pest populations get out of balance, growers will try various options such as insect predators, mating disruption, traps and barriers. If these fail, the certifier may grant permission to apply botanical or other non-persistent pesticides from the USDA National List of Approved Substances under restricted conditions. Botanicals are derived from plants and are broken down quickly by oxygen and sunlight.

The application of potentially harmful, long-lasting pesticides and fertilizers are not allowed in organic agriculture. The EPA considers 60% of all herbicides, 90% of all fungicides, and 30% of all insecticides as potentially cancer-causing."

Organic farmers can use both synthetic and natural kinds of pesticides —with approval under the USDA Organic Act. Many are harmless, yet others may raise eyebrows. To find out more specific information would require knowledge of the grower, as well as more detailed research on particular products allowed by the USDA (https://www.ams.usda.gov/about-ams/programs-offices/national-organic-program).

Glycemic Load vs. Glycemic Index

To measure the effect of food on blood sugar, scientists developed the glycemic index for foods. The index uses 50 grams of pure glucose as the number to which all other foods are measured. Scientists measured how quickly and how high blood sugar rose in reaction to eating the various foods tested. Glucose gets a score of 100 on the glycemic index and is the high mark (0 being the low). All foods measured are in 50-gram portions. So, eating foods with a low glycemic index (between 0-55 = low, 56-69 = medium and 70+ high) helps you avoid harmful blood sugar swings. Food manufacturers market some of their products as low-glycemic (or low GI); but this is misleading, since portion size is not taken into consideration.

We find problems in simply using the glycemic index as your guide. The first problem is the fixed portion size of 50 grams. When it comes to blood sugar issues, portion size is very important. If you look at the glycemic index, you will find that spaghetti pasta is listed as a moderate GI food; and carrots rank as high on the GI. Technically, this is accurate. However, no one eats only 50 grams, or one cup, of cooked of spaghetti noodles. Most people eat 2-3 cups for dinner, and that doubles or triples the index measure. Therefore, portion size of spaghetti pasta tells us that it is a VERY HIGH GI food. In terms of carrots, the equivalent of 50 grams is eight or nine big carrots! Perhaps Bugs Bunny can handle this, but the average human being simply does not eat this many carrots in a meal. The usual portion size of one to three carrots places this healthy food in the low GI measurement. Sadly, many people have avoided carrots, thinking they are a high-sugar, unhealthy food.

The next problem with the glycemic index is that it only measures the effects on blood sugar when the particular food is eaten alone, not with other foods. When foods are eaten with other foods such as a healthy fat, you may see a lower rise in blood sugar than when that food alone is eaten. Therefore, while the glycemic index is a useful tool, it is not an accurate measure of the effect on your blood sugar regarding whether a food should be eaten.

The Glycemic Load (GL) is a more accurate measure of what may happen to your blood sugar when you eat a typical food portion. Finding information for the GL of foods is just as easy as finding the GI and we have links to guides in our Resource and Reference Guide. In the glycemic load charts, you will see the serving size of that food, and its glycemic load (0-9=low; 10-19 – medium; 20+ high); you can adjust your portion sizes accordingly. So, if you eat mostly medium to high glycemic load foods, you will increase your risk of sugar surges, insulin spikes and insulin resistance. We recommend you limit or avoid these foods. The good news is that after you spend some time concentrating on low GL foods, your insulin responses may normalize, your body will run more efficiently, and you can then incorporate medium GL foods from time to time.

FATTY ACIDS / FATS

There are 4 types of fatty acids: (1) saturated; (2) monounsaturated; (3) polyunsaturated; and (4) trans fats). They have different chemical structures. Saturated fat has what is known as zero double bonds, monounsaturated has one double bond, and polyunsaturated has more than one double bond. Trans fats are in a class of their own and are odd-shaped with double bonds on opposite sides of the fat chain from where they occur in naturally occurring fats. Your body does not recognize them.

It used to be that saturated fats were considered the bad guys. We were told they caused heart disease and vascular disease. That misinformation led to people eating lots of margarine and other trans fats, and eliminating healthy foods like some meats, coconut and eggs! Saturated fats are key fats that perform critical roles in our bodies: (a) they provide stiffness and structure to our cell membranes and tissues; (b) they strengthen our immune system and help cells communicate better; (c) they help with hormone production; (d) they help with your nervous system; (e) they suppress inflammation (yep – they don't cause it, they help it!); and (f) they provide the nutrients needed for good brain function.

Monounsaturated fats are good for you and include the fats from olive oil, nuts, and some fish. Eating monounsaturated fats greatly benefits your heart and cardiovascular system, and improves your cholesterol numbers, which then helps prevent blood clots and stroke. These fats are also rich in Vitamin E and other antioxidants, and they improve insulin sensitivity, which greatly reduce your risk for diabetes, cancers, and other autoimmune diseases

Omega-6 and Omega-3 fats are polyunsaturated, and are considered essential fats, meaning they are necessary for optimal body function/health, but our bodies do not make them; so, we must eat these nutrients or take them as supplements. Polyunsaturated fats are needed for good cellular, immune, and hormonal function. Your cell membranes are made up primarily from Omega-3 fats that regulate insulin function, inflammation, and neurotransmitters. Polyunsaturated oils include soybean oil, canola, safflower, sunflower, flax, and fish oils. But not all of these are good choices! Food sources of polyunsaturated fats are walnuts, sunflower seeds, sesame seeds, pumpkin seeds, chia seeds, and fish. It's important to understand that the processing or cooking of polyunsaturated or monounsaturated fats affects their ability to be healthy or unhealthy. High heat damages these fats. Because of this, beware of Canola oil. Besides being primarily a Genetically Engineered Product (GMO), it is touted as being healthy omega-3 oil, but unfortunately, its processing makes it very unhealthy.

Artificial trans fats consist of artery-clogging fat that is made from vegetable oils, chemicals, and harmful metals. Hydrogen is pumped into the mixture to solidify the fat – where the term "hydrogenated or partially hydrogenated" comes from. It creates a shelf-stable fat those producers of packaged, processed foods just love! Great for the shelf life – killer of your life! You should avoid trans fats completely.

Look for hidden trans fats in baked goods, snack foods, frozen meals, cooking sprays, fake butters, coffee creamers, pre-made frostings, and of course, fast foods. Anything that says, partially hydrogenated is a trans fat. And of note: if a product says "no trans fats," by law it can still contain up to 0.5 grams!

OMEGA-6 VS. OMEGA-3 FATTY ACIDS

Both omega-6 and omega-3 fats are essential to your body. You must consume them, as your body needs them since you cannot make them on your own. Omega-6 is an inflammatory fatty acid. Omega-3 is anti-inflammatory. The ratio of omega-6 to omega-3 is important. Back before the time of processed foods and processed oils, our bodies would typically maintain a nice healthy 1:1 ratio of omega-6 to omega-3. Now, a typical ratio of 4:1, maybe even higher! We are consuming way too much omega-6 from vegetable, corn and seed oils, processed meats, and packaged foods, and not enough omega-3 from wild-caught fatty fish, pastured organic eggs, fish oil, and grass-fed meats. When this ratio is off, your body suffers from the imbalance. We see depressed immune systems, weight gain, and systemic/silent inflammation! This promotes conditions such as cardiovascular disease, cancer, and autoimmune diseases, to name a few.

Getting your body back in balance is very important, so eating fewer omega-6 fats and more omega-3 will enhance your health greatly. The best sources of omega-3 in your diet will be from wild-caught fatty fish like salmon, sardines and mackerel; high-quality fish oil supplements; pastured, organic eggs, and grass-fed meat (and if you so choose, grass-fed dairy). A whole host of diseases will be avoided or improved upon, and your brain will function optimally! Adequate levels of omega-3 fatty acids also improve depression and other depressive disorders. Fish oil becomes your Prozac!

When trying to consume more omega-3, note the two important types of omega-3 fatty acids, EPA and DHA. These are natural anti-inflammatory agents, playing a key role in many functions such as brain health, heart health, cancer protection, Alzheimer's disease protection, and much more.   EPA and DHA are found in the animal foods and supplements listed above. It is important to make sure that your high-quality fish oil supplement contains generous amounts of these two nutrients!

ANTIOXIDANTS

Antioxidants are substances that neutralize free radicals in our bodies.

Anti-:   (against, prevents, makes neutral)
Oxidant :   (to combine with oxygen)
Antioxidant: (to counter-act, go against oxidation).

We usually think of oxygen in terms of something good, right? For example, we need to breathe oxygen to live! Well, sometimes, our bodies can have too much oxidation on the cellular level, meaning our cells combine with oxygen; that combination produces particles called free radicals.

Free radicals are incomplete particles looking to get completed, like lonely little critters looking for a friend to grab onto. When they find a healthy cell or tissue to grab onto, then that cell or tissue is not whole anymore, and it looks for healthy cells or tissue to grab onto…and on and on. This causes those good cells and tissues to deteriorate or break down and become unhealthy cells and tissue. Antioxidants to the rescue! Antioxidants neutralize, or counteract, the bad stuff that the free radicals are causing. Many fruits and veggies are very high in antioxidants, and are our bodies' superheroes.

These superhero fruits and veggies (and other foods high in antioxidants) help your kidneys function well, protect your liver, help you age well, prevent wrinkles, support your immune system, help you sleep better, breathe better, keep you leaner, help your eyesight, your brain function, your digestion, and basically help keep you very healthy.

Some of the best fruits and veggies you can eat are on this list: acai', raisins, cherries, blueberries, blackberries, cranberries, garlic, kale, strawberries, cloves, spinach, broccoli, raspberries, coconut, chia seeds, and pumpkin seeds. And you may be thankful to know that dark chocolate is also a great antioxidant!

MICROBIOTA AND PROBIOTICS

Your GI (gastrointestinal) tract performs the essential functions of breaking down the foods we consume for nutrition, and preventing harmful substances from being absorbed into our bodies. Our GI tract relies upon a very complex ecosystem of bacteria, or microbiota (up to 10,000 different species of bacterial cells that make up more than 90% of the total cells in the human body). Every person has a unique flora system that starts at birth and changes over one's lifetime.

Normal gut flora supports a variety of intestinal functions, including production of digestive enzymes, which help with absorption of nutrients, and the support and stimulation of the immune system. It is estimated that 80% of our immune response is located in our intestinal tract. The beneficial bacteria residing in our guts work to prevent harmful bacteria from colonizing and taking up all of the space. They also produce a variety of substances that can inhibit, or even kill, potentially harmful bacteria. Our good bacteria also stimulate the secretion of IgA (immunoglobulin A), which serves on the first line of defense against infection, allergies, and inflammation.

Aging, poor nutrition, antibiotics, environmental toxins, stress, and antacids are a few of things that cause our delicate system of microbiota to get way out of balance. Through poor nutrition, we essentially starve our good bacteria of the nutrients they need, and constantly feed our bad bacteria the food they need – sugar! And to make matters worse, many develop a condition known as leaky gut, which causes gas, bloating, cramps, food sensitivities, joint pain, autoimmune disease, and skin rashes.

Leaky gut is defined as increased intestinal permeability or intestinal hyper-permeability. This happens when tight junctions in the gut, which control what passes through the lining of the small intestine, don't work properly. This can lead to substances leaking into the bloodstream, which causes the body to attack these foreign invaders and thus, the symptoms above begin. People with celiac disease and Crohn's disease experience this, but many others experience these symptoms as well.

Probiotics to the rescue! Probiotics are friendly bacteria that have beneficial effects on health. Probiotics modify the gut flora by replacing harmful microorganisms with useful microorganisms. Probiotic = for life.

Fermented foods are excellent sources of probiotic. Think sauerkraut, kimchi, fermented pickles, raw coconut yogurt, and coconut keifer. Since it's not that easy to get enough of these foods in our daily diet, using a high-quality probiotic supplement may be your best bet. Many people benefit greatly from the daily use of good probiotics and in time, begin to feel relief from some of the symptoms of an unbalanced gut.

In looking for a high-quality probiotic supplement, it is important to use a product that has a high culture count. This refers to the total amount of bacteria per serving. Look for a probiotic supplement with a minimum of 15 billion cultures in a single capsule. The number of strains is important too. Your probiotic supplement should include at least ten different strains of bacteria clinically proven to benefit optimal health. Look for high amounts of bifidobacteria for the large intestine (colon), and lactobacilli to support the small intestine. Other important criteria include finding a reputable manufacturer. Look for products manufactured by well-trusted companies with a good history of clinical evidence that their product works well, and also look for good reviews by users.

There are many excellent probiotic products on the market today. We list several in our Resource and Reference Guide that meet the criteria we have set forth.

FIBER

Another important element to a healthy digestive tract is fiber. Fiber is the substance typically found in fruits, vegetables, and grains that our bodies do not digest. Fiber actually passes quickly through your digestive tract, mostly intact, and it is not broken down like other foods. The fact that fiber is mostly left intact is a good thing because it creates bulk, which aids in moving stool and harmful waste through the digestive tract. Without enough fiber in your diet, you will experience irregularity, constipation, and sluggishness. Insufficient fiber can also increase your risk of colon cancer, as well as other serious health issues. Other health benefits of fiber include reducing the incidence of heart disease, lowering cholesterol, lowering blood pressure, stabilizing glucose levels, reducing systemic inflammation, and even aiding in weight loss.

There are two kinds of fiber: soluble and insoluble. We need both types. According to the Mayo Clinic, "Soluble fiber *dissolves* with water and creates a gel-like substance in your digestive tract, slowing digestion." To help lower and manage good blood cholesterol, soluble fiber attaches to cholesterol particles, taking them out of the body. And, since soluble fiber is not absorbed well, it slows the absorption of sugar, decreasing blood sugar spikes that put you at risk for type II diabetes or heart disease. Soluble fiber also soaks up water as it passes through your system, helping you stay regular and preventing both constipation and diarrhea. Examples of soluble fiber include apples, blueberries, citrus fruits, oats or oat bran, peas, rice bran, legumes/beans. Most fiber supplements also consist of soluble fiber.

Insoluble fiber retains more of its own form (does not turn to gel) and adds bulk to your digestive tract to keep things moving quickly. Insoluble fiber is found in the seeds and skin of plants, so always eat your peels. Insoluble fiber plays a key role in weight loss and weight management because it gives a sense of fullness which helps eliminate hunger pains. Examples of insoluble fiber include vegetables such as broccoli, cabbage, carrots, asparagus, brussels sprouts; and fruits such as raspberries and strawberries; nuts and seeds; and grains such as whole wheat, rye, and their brans.

According to the *Mayo Clinic*, we should be eating anywhere from 20 to 38 grams of fiber a day. The good news is that if you follow The Exercise Coach® Nutrition Playbook™ and eat foods listed on the Eat Daily and Eat Often lists, you will be just fine!

Food Allergies, Intolerance, and Sensitivities

Sometimes, even the most nutritious foods can be harmful to people who are allergic, intolerant, and/or sensitive to that food.

A food allergy is an abnormal response to a food, triggered by the body's immune system. In terms of this guide's discussion, an actual allergy is where the body produces a specific type of antibody, called immunoglobulin E (IgE). The binding of IgE antibodies to specific molecules in a food triggers the immune response. The response can range from mild to severe, and in rare cases, it can be associated with the severe and life-threatening reaction called anaphylaxis. If you suspect that you have a food allergy, it is extremely important for you to work with your healthcare professional to learn what foods are causing your allergic reaction.

Intolerance to certain foods can be similar to an allergy in terms of symptoms produced, but it does not involve the IgE antibodies. We are all bio-individual, and some of us simply cannot tolerate particular foods that others have no issue with. Common food intolerances include: lactose intolerance (the inability to process lactose, the sugar in milk, because the enzyme lactase is not being produced); gluten intolerance (similar to celiac disease, an autoimmune disorder which manifests as a negative reaction to the consumption of gluten); and food additive intolerance (reactions to food additives like MSG, sulfites, and food dye). While these are not true food allergies, they often produce terrible symptoms.

Food sensitivities are more controversial because they are not as easy to diagnose as a true IgE food allergy, or even food intolerance. And, to make things even more confusing, we can be sensitive to a food at some point in our lives, and not at another point. The very best way we can determine whether we have food sensitivity is through an elimination diet of that food (i.e. taking that food out of your diet for at least 4 weeks, then adding it back in to see if any reaction occurs). There are also food sensitivity tests that look for the presence of IgG antibodies. Many people have food sensitivities. The most common are dairy, wheat, eggs, nightshades (tomatoes, bell peppers, potatoes & eggplant), gluten, citrus, yeast, legumes, artificial sweeteners and food enhancers. Food sensitivities are important to uncover because they create an overworked immune system and lead to inflammation, digestive distress including leaky gut syndrome, weight gain, and other illnesses.

In discussing food sensitivities it is important to mention a term you may have come across: FODMAP, an acronym for **F**ermentable **O**ligo-, **D**i-, **M**onosaccharides **A**nd **P**olyols. These are complex names for a type of carbohydrate found in food that are sometimes poorly absorbed in the small intestine. When this occurs, these molecules act as a food source to the bacteria that live in the large intestine. The bacteria then digest/ferment these FODMAPs and can cause symptoms of irritable bowel syndrome (IBS). Symptoms include abdominal bloating and distension, excessive flatulence, abdominal pain, nausea, changes in bowel habits (diarrhea, constipation, or a combination of both), and other gastrointestinal symptoms. A few examples of food sources for each of the FODMAPs are listed below. The list is not complete and a great book is cited in our Resource and Reference Guide for further study. If you are experiencing symptoms of IBS, it may be beneficial to do an elimination diet of some of these foods as well.

- **Excess Fructose:** honey, apples, mangos, pears, watermelon, high-fructose corn syrup.
- **Fructans:** globe or Jerusalem artichokes, garlic (in large amounts), leeks, brown, white, or Spanish onions, onion powder, spring onions (white part), shallots, wheat (in large amounts), rye (in large amounts), barley (in large amounts), inulin/fructo-oligosaccharides (FOS).
- **Lactose:** milk, ice cream, custard, dairy desserts, condensed and evaporated milk, milk powder, yogurt, soft unripened cheeses (e.g. ricotta, cottage, cream, mascarpone).
- **Galacto-oligosaccharides (GOS):** legume beans (e.g. baked beans, kidney beans, bortolotti beans), lentils, chickpeas
- **Polyols:** apples, apricots, avocado, cherries, nectarines, pears, plums, prunes, mushrooms, sorbitol, mannitol, xylitol, maltitol, and isomalt.

Genetically Modified Organisms (GMO's)

GMOs ("genetically modified organisms") are living organisms whose genetic material has been artificially manipulated in a laboratory through genetic engineering, or GE. This relatively new science creates combinations of plant, animal, bacteria and viral genes that do not occur in nature or through traditional crossbreeding methods. GMOs were created to enhance growth and efficiency of plants (higher crop yields); increase resistance to pathogens, drought, bugs, and pesticides; to control viability of plants; and to increase nutritional content.

The big question is, are GMO foods safe? Most developed nations do not consider GMOs to be safe. In more than 60 countries around the world, including Australia, Japan, and all of the countries in the European Union, there are significant restrictions or outright bans on the production and sale of GMOs. In the U.S., the government has approved GMOs based on studies conducted by the same corporations that created them and profit from their sale. In addition, many studies have linked GMOs with a rise in food allergies, serious organ damage, nervous system disorders and even certain types of cancer. But the bottom line for many opposed to GMOs (including The Exercise Coach®) is that without enough research, there's simply no way to tell *how* harmful GMOs are. So it is a choice as to whether you believe it is a risk worth taking.

Increasingly, Americans are taking matters into their own hands and choosing to opt out of the GMO experiment. But it's not easy! Unfortunately, even though polls consistently show that a significant majority of Americans want to know if the food they're purchasing contains GMOs, this information is still being kept from the public in the U.S. Therefore, it's not a matter of checking food labels because that may not tell you. One way to know for sure is to purchase 100% certified organic food, which cannot include any GMOs. The second way is to look for the Non-GMO Project seal.

About 80% of processed foods in the U.S. contain GMOs. Currently the highest-risk crops are soy, alfalfa, canola, corn, cotton, papaya, sugar beets and zucchini. However, many other common crops may be genetically modified as well. The term *Frankenfoods* has come about because of the similarity of how Frankenstein was created – through piecing together lots of different organisms. On the horizon is the first genetically engineered animal: an Atlantic salmon that grows twice as fast as natural salmon, thanks to the insertion of genes from Chinook salmon and eelpout (an eel-like fish). Fortunately some retailers such as Whole Foods, Trader Joe, Walmart, Safeway, Kroger, Costco, and others will not be selling this product. In fact, Whole Foods is the first store to offer 100% GMO transparency for all products, by 2018. Hopefully others will follow suit.

Seafood: How to pick your seafood wisely

Seafood is an excellent protein source; however, not all fish are created equal. Some fish contain contaminants or are farmed using unhealthy methods. And even in the wild, many fish are high-risk when it comes to their mercury content.

The Exercise Coach® Nutrition Playbook™ recommends wild-caught, fatty fish that is high in omega-3 fatty acids. It would be beneficial to eat one of these choices at least two times per week to supply a generous amount of omega-3 fatty acids. Optimal choices are wild-caught salmon, anchovies, sardines, mackerel, lake and rainbow trout, black cod, and herring.

Purchasing seafood can be complicated, but no need to worry; the Seafood Watch Group of the Monteray Bay Aquarium has made it easy. The organization's website teaches you all you need to know about making excellent choices, including information about sustainable fishing techniques, and how the ocean's ecosystem can be protected. To help you make the best and healthiest choices in your area, download their free app, Seafood Watch, or print off one of their pocket-buying guides (See The Exercise Coach® Resource and Reference Links page 111).

The Exercise Coach® Supplement Guide

When it comes to nutritional supplements, we at The Exercise Coach® are truly fans! In today's world, you could probably be the world's best eater (organic, home-grown, non-GMO, pastured, grass-fed, wild, etc.), but you still would lack nutrients in your body for several good reasons. First, the soil today has been depleted of nutrients due to intensive modern agricultural practices, so foods grown in today's soil do not contain the micronutrients they once used to. Next, we have a large decrease in the diversity of plants consumed, and an increased exposure to food and environmental toxins that are harming our bodies. Finally, our lives are much more stress-filled, we are working longer, we are sleeping fewer hours per night, and we seem to get sick more often. This leads to the overuse of antibiotics, lack of sleep/exhaustion, and less time to be calm and quiet and enjoy nature. We don't even enjoy the sun like we used to due to concerns about skin cancer, so we miss out on our much-needed Vitamin D.

Ideally we would get all of the necessary nutrients from the food we eat, but that is not possible in today's world. Although supplementation is optional, The Exercise Coach® recommends adding nutrients to the diet that are beneficial and will aid general health. The following supplements are recommended by Dr. Mark Hyman, M.D., Director of The Center for Function Medicine, Cleveland Clinic. For some of our favorite sources and brands, check the Resource and Reference Links, page 112.

- High-quality multivitamin and multimineral supplement. This should include the majority of vitamins, antioxidants, and minerals you need to keep your body functioning well.
- One to two Grams of purified pharmaceutical-grade fish oil (EPA/DHA). This reduces overall inflammation, helps with insulin control and blood sugar balance, is a heart disease preventative, and a superfood for your brain.
- 2000-5000 iu of Vitamin D3. Up to 80% of the population is deficient in this important vitamin, yet it plays an incredibly important role in your overall health. It's best to get a vitamin D blood test to check your levels, use higher supplementation until you reach optimal levels, and then reduce to maintenance levels. (Studies have shown that our bodies absorb 32% more D3 when supplements are taken with a meal containing a fat).
- CoQ10 – This is beneficial for your heart and is a critical nutrient for turning food into energy inside of your cells.
- Magnesium (glycinate or malate) – Many people are deficient in this mineral as well. Magnesium improves sleep, reduces anxiety and muscle cramps, and helps control blood sugar. Please check with your doctor before supplementing if you have kidney issues).

- High-Quality Probiotics – Probiotics populate your gut with necessary healthy flora. This in turn reduces inflammation, gas and bloating, improves digestion, and helps heal leaky gut syndrome.
- Vitamin C – A good quality buffered product will help with detoxification, improve your immune system, and help with constipation.

While there are many other wonderful supplements that are specific to needs you may have, above is a general list for anyone who wishes to have good health. For specific dosages, nutrient needs, or deficiencies, please see a qualified nutritionist, physician, or health expert specializing in vitamins and supplementation.

The 30-Day Metabolic Comeback Challenge™

This can change your life! Why? Because during this challenge, you will not only change the way you are eating, you will change the way you look and feel! And, for many, you may improve long-term health indicators like body weight, cholesterol levels, blood sugar levels, and inflammation levels? YES – in just 30 days!

WE CHALLENGE YOU! DO YOU ACCEPT?

At The Exercise Coach®, studios hold 30-Day Metabolic Comeback Challenge™ contests several times each year. This is a wonderful opportunity to join with others participating and potentially be the winner! But don't let the lack of an organized contest stop you! A personal, 30-Day Metabolic Comeback Challenge™ can take place any time. Your Exercise Coach team would love to help you get started, guide you along the way, and cheer you on to victory!

The 30-Day Metabolic Challenge™ is a 30-day period where The Food Villains are eliminated completely. We want to take out any potential inflammatory food, any food with a high likelihood to cause allergy or sensitivity, and all processed and fake foods. And, all sugars! Many symptoms you experience day to day could be linked to what you eat. Many who eat "healthy" find that eliminating these culprits clears things up. You may experience what others have: weight loss, more energy, better sleep, lack of sugar cravings, better digestion, better emotional health, fewer aches and pains, clearer skin, weakened seasonal allergies, less gas and bloating… and the list goes on.

THE CHALLENGE IS ON!

WHAT FOODS ARE ELIMINATED?

Now that you have accepted the challenge, here is the list of prohibited foods during the 30-Day time frame. For a complete list of what these include, please refer back to the Super Villain sections in the beginning of this guide, page 6.

- Super Villain #1 – All forms of Sugar
  - All forms of natural sugars.
  - No fruit juices or coconut water or fruits preserved in juices or syrups

- Super Villain #2 – All grains and starches
  - No white starches (white potatoes, Yukon gold, red, fingerling)
- Super Villain #3 – Dairy products
- Super Villain #4 – Legumes and Soy
- Super Villain #5 – Artificial sweeteners, MSG, carrageenan, artificial colors
- Super Villain #6 – Processed Meals (anything in a bag or box, or processed ingredients)
- Super Villain #7 – Alcoholic Beverages (or cooking with them)
- Gluten. Gluten lurks in many foods, most of which are not allowed during the challenge. Be careful if gluten is included in your vinegar, your unsweetened condiments, etc.
- Bad Fats/unhealthy Oils. This includes corn oils, peanut oils, soybean oil, vegetable oil, canola oil, trans-fats, margarines, any nut or seed butters with added sugar, peanut butter.
- Some Condiments. This includes any that have sugar or unhealthy oils, or other "off limit" ingredients. (Make your own with our recipes or search out those that truly do not contain any of these harmful ingredients).

WHAT WILL I EAT FOR 30 DAYS?

We have made it super easy for you to shop and decide what to eat! Our handout, What Should Be On My Plate is included in this guide, and is also available at your Exercise Coach® studio. Take a photo on your smart phone and have it with you at all times! We have also assembled a 30-day sample meal plan that you can use in its entirety, or simply be inspired with a few dishes. Your choices will include items listed earlier in the guide, under What Shall We Eat, page 19.

- Good source protein (beef, poultry, game, fish, eggs, supplemental)
- Plenty of vegetables (includes starchy, colorful veggies such as sweet potatoes or squash)
- Legumes (only green beans, snap peas and snow peas since they are more "pod" than "bean" and have many healthy benefits)
- Fruit (includes starchy fruits like bananas or papaya)
- Healthy fats (olive oils, coconut oil, avocado oil, avocado, nuts, seeds, nut milk, nut butter, olives, organic butter/ghee)
- Spices and seasonings, including good high-quality sea salt
- Purified water (plain, infused, sparkling, mineral), unsweetened tea, unsweetened coffee), unsweetened nut milks
- Smoothies (protein, veggie)
- Condiments (dressings, vinegars, guacamole, ketchup, mayo, mustard, salsa, relish, etc.) that do not contain sugar or artificial ingredients
- Small amounts of stevia or sugar alcohols (xylitol, erythritol, etc.)
- *Note: For vegetarians or vegans, eating legumes and using supplemental protein may be necessary if eggs and/or fish are not options.*

THE METABOLIC COMEBACK

During the 30 Day Challenge, eat ONLY these foods. Ongoing, choose these 80% of the time.

WHAT SHOULD BE ON MY PLATE?

HIGH QUALITY PROTEIN

Organic, Grass-Fed, or Free-Range best, but not required. Eat 1-2 palm sized, and palm thick portions. For eggs, eat 2-4.

- BEEF
- CHICKEN
- FISH
- PORK
- GAME MEATS
- EGGS
- COACH FUEL – DF
- COACH BARS - DF

VEGETABLES

Organic when possible (especially those listed on the EWG "dirty dozen" list). Eat generous portions! Try new varieties.

ARTICHOKE	CUCUMBER	PEPPERS
ARUGULA	EGGPLANT	PUMPKIN
ASPARAGUS	GARLIC	RADISH
BEETS	GREEN BEANS	SNOW PEAS
BOK CHOY	GREENS	SPINACH
BROCCOLI & RABE	JICAMA	SQUASH
BRUSSELS SPROUTS	KALE	SWEET POTATO
CAULIFLOWER	KOHLRABI	SWISS CHARD
CABBAGE	LETTUCE	TOMATO
CARROTS	MUSHROOMS	TURNIP
CELERY	ONIONS	WATERCRESS
CELERY ROOT	PARSNIPS	ZUCCHINI

FRUITS

Organic when possible (especially those listed on the EWG "dirty dozen"). 1 serving per meal.

	BLACKBERRIES	GRAPES	MELONS	PEARS	STRAWBERRIES
	BLUEBERRIES	KIWI	NECTARINE	PINEAPPLE	TANGERINES
APPLES	CHERRIES	LEMONS	ORANGES	PLUM	WATERMELLON
APRICOTS	DATES/FIGS	LIMES	PAPAYA	POMEGRANITE	DRIED FRUIT
BANANAS	GRAPEFRUIT	MANGO	PEACHES	RASPBERRIES	(SMALL QUANTITIES ONLY)

For healthy, delicious recipes following these guidelines, visit our website: www.exercisecoach.com/resources/nutrition OR our Pinterest Page: http://www.pinterest.com/exercisecoach OR our Facebook page: https://www.facebook.com/theexercisecoach. New recipes added each week!

(OVER)

HEALTHY FATS

Choose 1-2 fat sources per meal.

OILS – 1-2 THUMB SIZE PORTIONS

ORGANIC BUTTER	COCONUT OIL
AVOCADO OIL	OLIVE OIL
SESAME OIL (COLD)	PALM OIL
FLAXSEED OIL (COLD)	GHEE
NUT OILS (COLD)	DUCK FAT

AVOCADO – ½ - 1 PER MEAL

COCONUT MILK – ¼ - ½ CAN

OLIVES – 1-2 OPEN HANDFULS

COCONUT SHREDDED – 1-2 HANDFULS

NUTS/SEEDS – 1 SMALL HANDFUL

BEVERAGES

WATER

FRUIT/HERB/VEGGIE INFUSED WATER

SPARKLING OR MINERAL WATER

COFFEE (UNSWEETENED)*

TEA (UNSWEETENED)*

COCONUT MILK

GREEN SMOOTHIES (UNSWEETENED)*

COACH FUEL–DF SMOOTHIES (UNSWEETENED)*

ALMOND MILK

ICED TEA (UNSWEETENED)

*PURE STEVIA ALLOWED IN SMALL AMOUNTS

SPICES / SEASONINGS

BASIL	CILANTRO	GARLIC	NUTMEG	SAVORY
BAY LEAVES	CLOVE	GINGER	OREGANO	SPEARMINT
BLACK PEPPER	CINNAMON	HORSERADISH	PAPRIKA	TARRAGON
CARDAMOM	COCOA (100%)	LEMONGRASS	PARSLEY	THYME
CAYENNE	CUMIN	MARJORAM	PEPPERMINT	TURMERIC
CHILI POWDER	CURRY	MINT	ROSEMARY	VANILLA
CHIVES	DILL	MUSTARD	SAGE	VINEGAR

CONDIMENTS

Home-made only. Unsweetened*

ASIAN DRESSING	PICKLES/RELISH (UNSWEETENED)*
BBQ SAUCE	
GUACAMOLE	SALSA
KETCHUP	VINAIGRETTE
MAYO	
MUSTARD (MOST STORE BOUGHT OK)	

*PURE STEVIA ALLOWED IN SMALL AMOUNTS

EWG'S DIRTY DOZEN 2016

Shoppers Guide to Pesticides in Produce

APPLES	SPINACH
CELERY	STRAWBERRIES
CHERRIES	SWEET BELL PEPPERS
CHERRY TOMATOES	TOMATOES
CUCUMBERS	PLUS +
GRAPES	HOT PEPPERS
NECTARINES	KALE/COLLARDS
PEACHES	

ENVIRONMENTAL WORKING GROUP

PREPARING FOR THE 30-DAY CHALLENGE

You wouldn't take a big vacation without planning your itinerary, your hotels, your transportation, and your finances. In the same way, we think you should plan ahead for your 30-Day Metabolic Comeback Challenge!™ It's a big change, and a little planning will go a long way toward success. During this time, you will make over your kitchen and pantry, plan your meals for the next 30 days, shop for items that can be frozen or that do not perish quite so fast, prepare your shopping list of fresh foods in advance, get some initial measurements recorded (body weight, body fat, waist and thigh circumference), and get your mind geared up for this exciting time!

Kitchen and Pantry Makeover

To ensure success, it is best to clear your kitchen and pantry of foods that are not allowed during The 30-Day Metabolic Comeback™. We especially recommend clearing those that may be more enticing to you. Clear out foods such as those that contain sugar (cookies, cakes, other bakery items, candy); natural sweeteners (refined sugar, honey, agave syrup, maple syrup, etc.); snack chips; sodas and sugary drinks including fruit juice; milk and dairy products except organic butter or clarified butter/ghee; flours; breads; grains; processed boxed or bagged meals; margarine; artificial sweeteners and any products containing them; and corn, vegetable, and soybean oils (and any other hydrogenated or refined oils). Of course, if some of these items are on the Eat Sometimes or Eat Rarely list (page 57) and you wish to keep them for future use, you can simply put them to the side, out of sight, for 30 days.

Meal Planning

Don't find yourself in a food emergency! Planning your meals for The 30-Day Metabolic Comeback™ will be one of the most important things you can do. That's not to say you cannot still participate "on the fly." By all means, participate and plan as you get under way! While this 30-day period is intended to reset your metabolism, and reset your mind on how to eat, it is also a time to reset how you plan and choose what you eat for life. Nothing is more empowering than choosing the right fuel for your body and being in control of your health as much as you possibly can be!

On page 61 you will find a sample menu for the 30 days. While the menu is not necessarily meant to be followed to the letter (although you may choose to do that), it is a wonderful guide to the possibilities that exist with the foods you are allowed to eat. Choose some of the menu items or choose everything on the menu – the choice is yours. In addition, The Exercise Coach® website (www.exercisecoach.com), along with The Exercise Coach® Pinterest page is filled with recipes that are approved for the 30-Day Metabolic Comeback.™ If you are game, create your own 30-day menu! In our Resource and Reference Guide we have included a Meal Planning for the 30-Day

Metabolic Comeback™ worksheet. Copy as many sheets as you need and begin your planning. And remember, you can easily think of breakfasts in terms of smoothies, which makes planning that meal a breeze!

Food Journal

Included in this guide is The Exercise Coach® Food Journal (page 79). We encourage you to use it. It is well established that recording what you eat will keep you on track. For the 30 days, your meal planning should do that for you, so this guide is useful if you wish to see exactly what you ate, and notice any inconsistencies, any foods that still gave you trouble, and what combinations worked best for you. An ongoing food journal will help you stay within your means. When you record what you eat, you are not likely to over-eat, or eat too many foods that are on the Eat Rarely list, and you will notice foods that give you any issues as you write down any reactions in the notes section. A food journal truly can provide you with a thorough understanding of your own eating habits, as well as help you cultivate and maintain healthy-eating habits.

Grocery Lists and Shopping

Now comes the fun part! After you have your meals all planned or at least have a grasp of what you are allowed to eat, you get to make your list and shop! There's something quite rewarding about filling your cart with healthy, whole-food items. Remember, we have made this very easy. There are two ways to complete your list. The first is to look at your completed meal plan and write down the ingredients you need to purchase for week #1. The second, if you are not planning ahead, is to take the What Should Be On My Plate handout to the store with you, and purchase items in each category that you do not have in your refrigerator or pantry. Purchase items you believe you will use and that you enjoy eating. But remember, it's important to be open to trying new varieties of vegetables in a variety of colors, as well as some fruits you may not typically eat. Each week of the challenge, continue to shop a week ahead so that you are fully prepared. And remember to stock those healthy snack and beverage options. You don't want to find yourself hungry or thirsty and reaching for an unapproved snack or beverage. (Check out our Healthy Snack blog in The Exercise Coach® Resource and Reference Guide, page 100).

Dining out During your Challenge

Eating out on the 30-Day challenge requires effort because you will be hard-pressed to find choices that fulfill the requirements. Restaurants are notorious for adding hidden sugar and/or dairy. And, it's impossible to know whether additives are a part of your nice-looking meal. If you must eat out (and many who travel do), choose a restaurant ahead of time that you believe will fit your needs. Look up their menu in advance and even call to ask questions. Ask what type of oil may be used in the meal preparation, and whether they can substitute for you. You can also ask about added sugars or other hidden ingredients. Most restaurants offer gluten free options so it's best to start there. When in doubt, salads are always an option, especially at fast-food restaurants. Ask for one with no sugar, and ask for olive oil, vinegar and lemon to use for dressing (or bring your own). You can also count on breakfast restaurants for a nice omelet. Just ask that yours be prepared with olive oil and without any added dairy ingredients. You may add a side of veggies prepared in the same olive oil or steamed. If you choose Mexican food, order the fajitas, ask for olive oil, and eat the meat with plenty of veggies. Skip the sides and use lettuce as your tortilla. If push comes to shove and there is no choice, don't worry about the type of oil they are using or things you cannot control, and eat the food that is allowed on the 30-Day Metabolic Comeback Challenge.™

Getting Measured

Prior to beginning your 30-Day Metabolic Comeback,™ your Certified Exercise Coach will record certain measurements. While people's numbers vary greatly over the 30 days, you will see some improvement in some of the key areas of measurement, even in that short period of time! We hope this will encourage you to keep on keepin' on. The measurements most commonly recorded are body weight, body fat percentage, and lean body mass (muscle). In addition, you can have your circumference measured at your thigh, waist or any other location you may desire, as well as your height. Medical measurements such as blood pressure, resting heart rate, glucose & A1C, triglycerides, cholesterol, etc. are also wonderful to obtain from your doctor. Once you complete your 30 days, it will be important to remeasure within one to two days. If your goal is weight loss or an improvement in a health condition and you are going to continue onward for 60 or 90 days, etc., we highly recommend medical measurements. Our clients have heard this from many doctors: "whatever you are doing, keep doing it!"

Setting your mind on the goal

Like most athletes getting ready for a competition, mindset matters! Focus on the positive. Think about how you want to feel, ideally, and look toward that as a real possibility. Remind your Certified Exercise Coach, family and friends that you are about to take the challenge, and accept their encouragement. You can do this! And best of all, it's just 30 days.

EXPECTATIONS

The 30-Day Metabolic Comeback™ seeks to put you in an optimized hormonal state. We encourage you to follow the program to the letter; but, if you slip up a little along the way, you are always just one whole food meal away from a healthier hormonal state. So get back up and keep going. The Exercise Coach® is a guilt free encouragement zone!

Week 1

You may find that you feel worse during week 1. Don't worry; this is actually normal. It's evidence that many of the non-whole foods you eat create a dependency on them. This will pass and when it does, you will likely feel so good that you will not want to go back to unhealthy eating. Remember also to be kind to your brain during this change. Drink lots of fresh water, have a healthy snack if you feel a loss of energy, try to get at least 8 hours of sleep each night, and if possible, take five to ten minutes each day to sit quietly and breathe at a rate of six breaths per minute.

Last, don't beat yourself up if your workouts feel harder the first week. Your body is adjusting to new energy sources. Everyone gets an A for effort during their workouts this first week!

Week 2

Hopefully you will start to experience some of the great benefits in week 2: weight loss, better sleep, more energy, improved workout recovery, reduction in body ailments, and less stress.

The most important thing this week is to stick with it! There will be temptations. Don't give in. If you feel weak, eat more food! Remember, this is not a low calorie diet. At a meal, eat until you are comfortably full, and especially, eat more veggies and good fat. This is critical since your body needs the energy from the fat. And remember, snacks are optional. If you are eating correctly during your meals at this point, you may be able to skip at least one of your snacks each day. Our bodies are smart. They make us think we are hungry when in reality, we just have a craving. Learn your own body signals and stop being tricked into thinking you need food all the time.

Week 3

By week 3 you will be getting used to eating right. This is a time to be creative and try new foods. By week 3, your taste buds will be adjusting and you will rediscover all kinds of new and yummy flavors.

For some, you still may not be feeling as good as you think you should be, or losing weight as you had hoped (if that was your goal). We recommend you talk to your Exercise Coach about this. There's a good chance that others have also had the same experience and your coach can help with a solution. Perhaps your snacking habits need monitoring. Maybe you are not eating enough vegetables and fat. Perhaps the environmental toxins you still experience (detergents, cleaning products, lotions, etc.) are an inflammatory burden. Our 30-Day Metabolic Comeback Challenge™

is powerful, but 14-21 days just might not be quite enough time to undue the 20, 30, or 50+ years of battering we put our body through. Stay the course!

In this final week, you will be able to see the finish line! We truly hope you will feel great and experience noticeable changes in mood, energy, weight, and overall well-being.

Whether you follow the program perfectly or slip up again and again, the final week counts. It counts because you will cross the finish line. Over 30 days you will have begun creating new neural maps for healthy eating behavior. And, seeing the finish line makes everybody feel stronger! We want you to build momentum, and finish strong.

POST 30-DAY CHALLENGE

Congratulations! You have completed your 30-Day Metabolic Comeback Challenge.™ This was not easy and we are proud that you have taken this step toward better heath.

Now that you are eating better, feeling better, and looking better, what's next? We hope a return to your old habits is not the answer! Just because it is Day 31 does not mean you jump ship. For some, the results are amazing: (1) weight loss, (2) better sleep, (3) clearer skin, (4) reduction of headaches and stress, and (5) increased strength and overall health. Some may still crave poor choice foods, have a hard time with sleep, and simply not feel more energized. While that is not the typical response, it happens occasionally. Why? You have just put in an amazing 30 days of hard work, but 30 days might not be quite enough time to undue 20, 30, or 50+ years of poor nutrition. It may simply take more time! There is no magic number. For some it's 60 days, for others 120 days. If you do give yourself enough time, you will see and feel results!

If you are happy with your 30-day results, or want to be able to add in a few other food choices, we suggest adding those foods in slowly, one at a time. For example, if you have decided to add dairy, add in one dairy product for four days and see how you feel. See if you notice reactions of any kind with energy levels, headaches, allergies, or skin conditions. If all is fine, add in another dairy product for four more days, checking again for any reactions. After those eight days, perhaps you may want to add in a particular grain like steel cut oatmeal (we suggest starting with non-gluten grains). Again, add in for four days and note any reactions. It's suggested to continue this way until you add most of the food groups back in that you expect to eat. If you do notice a reaction, stop eating that food for a week and see if the reaction subsides. This method is really the best way to see how your body responds to foods. It will help you make better choices.

We hope you continue to center your eating around healthy, whole foods, and that your primary choices are those foods you eat during the 30-Day Metabolic Comeback Challenge.™ However, there are other foods that are on the <u>Eat Sometimes</u> or <u>Eat Rarely</u> list that you can choose from as well, as long as they do not become your primary food choices.

Life After The 30-Day Metabolic Comeback™

80/20 HEALTH FOR A LIFETIME PLAN™

Life after the 30-Day Metabolic Challenge™ can include a wide variety of foods. We know that variety is the spice of life, and everyone wants birthday cake and ice cream now and then. We recommend our guide, The 80/20 Health for a Lifetime Plan. Under this plan, you choose your foods from those allowed on the 30-Day Metabolic Comeback Challenge™ (those listed below on the Eat Daily and Eat Often lists) 80% of the time. The other 20% of the time choose foods from every other list (except the Never Eat list). Whether this is five days of exceptional eating (i.e. only those foods on the Eat Daily and Eat Often list) and two days of whatever you like from the other lists, or whether 80% of your daily intake is based on foods on the Eat Daily or Eat Often list, and 20% from the other lists, do your best to stick to healthy whole food eating! Basically, think of other foods as secondary to the foods you are allowed on the 30-Day Metabolic Comeback Challenge.™ You decide. It's your body; it's your health.

We have put together some lists to help you choose your foods over the period of a day, week, or month. If you choose to live on The 80/20 Health for a Lifetime Plan™, these lists will assist you in choosing those "20% of the time" foods that you may simply enjoy, but may not be the best choices in terms of good nutrition. Even if you are not making foods on the Eat Daily and Eat Often list your primary choices, these lists will help you see, over time, what category the choices you are making fall into. And, that may encourage you to choose less of those, and more of the healthier choices. Any food should be off your list if you are allergic or sensitive to it. And if you hope to lose more weight, eat foods other than those listed on the Eat Daily or Eat Often far less than 20% of the time until your desired weight is reached.

EAT DAILY

All foods and beverages allowed on the 30-Day Metabolic Comeback Challenge™ are included on the Eat Daily list. We believe you need to eat something from each major category, every single day, several times per day.

- Filtered water (preferably not from plastic bottles or plastic water coolers)
- Vegetables (wide variety of types and color)
- Good source protein (meat, fish, eggs, organic, pastured, free-range preferred)

- Healthy fats/oils (olive oil, avocado oil, organic coconut oil, sesame oil, flaxseed oil, organic butter or ghee, nut oils, MCT oil, duck fat, organic palm oil, coconut, olives)

EAT OFTEN

Foods on the Eat Often list do not have to be consumed daily, but should be a regular part of your weekly diet unless a medical reason exists that precludes you from eating that food.

- Fruits
- Nuts/seeds
- Spices and seasonings
- Unsweetened condiments / vinegars
- Coach Fuel™ shakes and green smoothies

EAT SOMETIMES

Foods on the Eat Sometimes list can be eaten up to three times per week, but are not necessary to your healthy diet (i.e. you can get the nutrients from the Eat Daily and Eat Often foods).

- Raw milk (only if you have ability to obtain from a great source you trust)
- Steel cut oatmeal
- Organic milk, cheese, sour cream, non-dessert dairy (grass fed preferred)
- Quinoa
- Brown rice
- Buckwheat
- Beans (properly soaked and prepared)
- Wine or alcoholic (unsweetened) beverage (if you are generally healthy)
- Coconut water *(choose low sugar, well-made products)*
- Desserts prepared with no sugars or flours (stevia o.k. as sweetener)

EAT RARELY

Foods on the Eat Rarely list can be eaten up to seven times per month, depending on your overall health and desired weight levels. These are foods that contain the Super Villain we have that love/ hate relationship with: Sugar! Eat foods on this list as rarely as possible.

- Cookies
- Cakes
- Candy

- Baked goods
- Bread
- Crackers
- White rice
- White potatoes
- Corn (organic) and organic corn products
- French fries
- Pizza
- Fast foods
- Other grains (and any food made from them)
- Processed foods (not those containing artificial ingredients, dyes, MSG, or trans-fats)
- Flours
- Pasta
- Chips, pretzels, other crunch snack foods
- Peanuts
- Dips
- Fruit juices
- Ice cream (*sorbet, gelato, etc.*)
- Sugary desserts
- Fruit juice (no extra sugar added)
- Soda (not diet, preferably those with stevia)
- Sugary alcoholic beverage (if generally healthy)
- Soy products (fermented types)
- Vegetable & seed oils (if other choices are not possible)

NEVER EAT

- Diet soda
- Artificial sweeteners (or any food made with them)
- MSG
- Carrageenan (contained in some nut milks and other products)
- Artificial colors, additives or fillers
- Trans-fats (or any foods made with them or in them)
- Soy (non-fermented types)

Now that you are well on your way to understanding what it takes to purify your eating, and in turn, gain control over your health, it's time we give a little attention to an area most of us probably take for granted: our hygiene products, and products we use in the home to keep our environment clean. It's ironic that most of what we use to keep our homes, clothing, and body clean are actually making us sick! Suzanne Somers explains in her book, <u>Tox-Sick, From Toxic to Not Sick,</u> that most of the cleaners and hygiene products we use contain harmful, harsh chemicals. These cause harmful side affects, some of which are allergic reactions, skin rashes, headaches, and even cancer! To find out about the products you use or may want to use, the Environmental Working Group (EWG) publishes a list of most common and specialty products, ranks them for overall safety, and allows you to read about each ingredient and its dangers. (See the link in The Exercise Coach® Resource and Reference Guide, pages 108 and 109).

According to the EWG, one out of every three chemical cleaning products contains ingredients that are known to cause human health or environmental problems. Yet the corporations making these products have no legal obligation to tell you that. Have you ever read your shampoo bottle? And cosmetics are a haven for toxins. Our skin is the largest organ in the body and our pores soak up everything, even pollutants in the air. And when you consider that most cosmetics are laden with plastic as a main ingredient, and many lipsticks with lead, it's time to rethink your makeup!

To begin your own chemical cleanup, we encourage you to take a look at the following products you may use and evaluate them for harsh chemicals and harmful ingredients, using the EWG's guide: laundry detergent, fabric softener, household cleaners, air fresheners, candles, dish soaps, hand soaps, body soaps and gels, deodorants, lotions and creams, cosmetics, hair sprays, shampoo and conditioners, toothpaste, mouthwashes, perfumes, etc. If the guide does not list your products, look up the ingredients from the product label.

While it is not possible to completely eliminate the toxic burden we are all under, we can do a lot to reduce it. Every time you use a product, ask yourself: "Is this full of chemicals? Is there a possible natural alternative?" The key is to become cognizant. Over time, you will at least gain control over the items you use in your own home.

The Exercise Coach® uses pure, organic cleaners and products in their studios. Don't be fooled by the myth that organic cleaners do not clean or disinfect like bleaches or other harmful chemicals. It's simply not true!

The Exercise Coach® Nutrition Playbook™ is touching on this subject briefly to encourage you to first, clean up your nutrition, and also clean up your personal environment. Here are a few recommendations from Suzanne Somers's book <u>Tox-Sick, From Toxic to Not Sick</u>:

a. Always read ingredients on what you buy, and if you do not recognize some, look them up and see if they have harmful properties
b. Look for ingredients derived from plants and minerals
c. Products containing petroleum-derived or petrochemical ingredients are a no-no
d. Look for the origin of a fragrance (natural or not)
e. Ingredients should be biodegradable
f. Products should not be animal tested
g. Products should be safe for septic systems
h. Products must not cause corrosion
i. Products must be free of known human carcinogens, mutagens, teratogens, and endocrine disruptors

We've listed a variety of sources for products in The Exercise Coach® Nutrition Playbook® Resource and Reference Guide. In addition, if you shop at Whole foods, you can buy anything tagged as a "Premium Product" with trust that it has already passed the rigorous standards equal to those we recommend. And remember, Grandma used to use safe, common household ingredients for many of her cleaning and hygiene needs (baking soda, vinegar, borax, soap, washing soda, cornstarch, lemon, etc.). If you are creative and enjoy your own little science project, check out some recipes in The Exercise Coach® Resource and Reference Guide, page 109.

The journey doesn't end here. Cleaning up your toxic world means replacing plastics in your home with glass, drinking water from your own filter and not out of a plastic bottle or jug, or standard water cooler, replacing cookware with safer types, using natural bug sprays, eliminating chemical pesticides and herbicides, growing your own vegetables organically, and the list goes on. The good news is, you don't have to be overwhelmed. This is a one-foot in front of the other journey. What we have observed is that once you become passionate about what you put in your body, you will slowly become passionate about what you put on and around your body as well. It's a process well worth the effort.

Worksheets, handouts, articles, books and websites,
including those used in the research for
this Playbook, that support facts or conclusions presented

Printable copies of the handouts and worksheets are available at
www.exercisecoach.com / password: **comeback30days#**

SAMPLE MENU FOR THE 30-DAY METABOLIC COMEBACK CHALLENGE™

A simple way to plan of each of your three meals is to choose a protein, one or two vegetables, a healthy fat, and your spices and seasonings. Then, you can choose to add a fruit to one meal perhaps, or use as a snack. In constructing your meals this way, you can look at the <u>What Should I Eat</u> guide and make your choices for each meal or snack. To make it even simpler, choose to have some form of Coach Fuel-DF™ Smoothie every day for one of your main meals.

Many of us desire more creativity in our meals and will combine the components in one casserole or overall recipe. The great news is that The Exercise Coach® has an extensive list of healthy breakfasts, smoothies, lunches, snacks, condiments, salads, dinners, sides, soups, and even desserts posted on The Exercise Coach® Pinterest and Facebook pages, and on our website (www.exercisecoach. com). We add to these weekly and indicate which are 30-Day Metabolic Comeback™ approved (or if not, how to make them that way). Listed below is a sample of a 30-day menu plan. Each recipe is 30-Day Metabolic Comeback™ approved, and every recipe marked with an asterisk (*) is located on The Exercise Coach® Pinterest page and website (www.exercisecoach.com).

Look over the menu a week ahead of time, and be sure you have the necessary ingredients. You can mix and match any way you like, but we recommend you try to use ingredients you purchase in multiple meals that week. Also, leftovers are great and as you will see in our 30-day sample plan, we spread out leftovers over a few days. Please note that some recipes need to be prepared in advance, and we have indicated this with the symbol (♦)

For portion sizes, refer back to the section about portion size, page 27. And remember, if you do not need a snack mid-morning or mid-afternoon, it's fine to skip it. While there are not rules regarding what time to eat, we recommend that you finish eating dinner before 7:00 p.m. so your body can digest your meal before bedtime.

DAY 1

Breakfast
>   Omelet with tomatoes, spinach, red bell pepper, onion

Snack
>   Almonds

Lunch
>   Tomato, cucumber & avocado salad*

Snack
>   Apple with almond butter

Dinner
>   Chicken and carrots with lemon butter sauce*

DAY 2

Breakfast
>   Coach Fuel™ green smoothie* (1 scoop Coach Fuel-DF™ with any veggie smoothie recipe)

Snack
>   ½ avocado with sea salt

Lunch
>   Slow cooker squash soup*◆
>   Raw apple slices

Snack
>   Raw medium cucumber or pickle

Dinner
>   Citrus salmon with broccoli* (omit sugar)

Day 3

Breakfast
>   Eggs over easy with garlic- sautéed spinach in olive oil
>   Slice of tomato & bell pepper

Snack
>   Plantain chips (Trader Joe's)

Lunch
>   Grilled chicken, seasoned to taste

Side salad with olive oil & vinegar
Snack
    Medium apple
Dinner
    Italian pot roast* (crockpot)◆

Day 4

Breakfast
    Coach Fuel-DF™ chocolate smoothie *(see recipe page 73)*
Snack
    ½ banana and a few plantain chips
Lunch
    Slow cooker squash soup* - *leftovers from Day 2*
Snack
    Hard-boiled egg ◆
Dinner
    Butternut squash chili with beef*◆ (no beans or dairy added)

Day 5

Breakfast
    Supreme egg loaf*◆   (1 lg. slice)
    Berries
Snack
    1 oz. of dark chocolate (no sugar added) and 1 oz. pistachios
Lunch
    Butternut squash chili with beef* - *leftovers from Day 4*
Snack
    Hard-boiled egg ◆
Dinner
    Italian pot roast* - *leftovers from Day 3*

Day 6

Breakfast
    Coach Fuel-DF™ smoothie* *(see recipe page 73)*
Snack
    RXBAR® of choice

Lunch

      Supreme egg loaf*◆   (1 lg. slice)

      One orange

Snack

      ½ avocado with sea salt

Dinner

      Ancho-rub flank steak w/ side of arugula & cherry tomato* (eliminate brown sugar)

Day 7

Breakfast

      Supreme egg loaf*◆   (1 lg. slice)

      Berries

Snack

      Raw carrots

Lunch

      Classic Cobb salad (no cheese added) *with homemade vinaigrette*◆

Snack

      Apple with almond butter

Dinner

      Cilantro lime chicken with avocado salsa*

Day 8

Breakfast

      Supreme egg loaf ◆

      Macadamia nuts

Snack

      Banana

Lunch

      Grilled chicken on greens with veggies of choice, homemade creamy avocado dressing*

Snack

      Hard-boiled egg ◆

Dinner

      Citrus salmon with broccoli*

      Raw carrots

Day 9

Breakfast

    Coach Fuel™ green smoothie*

Snack

    1 oz. of dark chocolate (no sugar added)

    Berries

Lunch

    Scrambled eggs with Exercise Coach homemade salsa *(see recipe page 74)*

Snack

    Almonds

Dinner

    Coach's lettuce wrap tacos *(see recipe page 74)*

    Exercise Coach salsa *(see recipe page 74)*

    Guacamole*

    Raw veggies

Day 10

Breakfast

    Two hard-boiled eggs ◆

    Cashews

Snack

    Apple slices with cashew or almond butter

Lunch

    Coach Fuel-DF™ chocolate smoothie* *(see recipe page 73)*

Snack

    ½ avocado with salt

Dinner

    Thai cashew chicken and mango salad

Day 11

Breakfast

    Coach Fuel™ green smoothie of choice*

Snack

    Pistachios and an orange

Lunch

Taco salad (use leftover taco meat from Day nine on top of chopped greens, with chopped mango, leftover guacamole,* and chopped tomato)

Snack

Raw celery sticks with nut butter

Dinner

Moroccan spiced pork chops with mashed sweet potatoes (substitute nut milk)*

Day 12

Breakfast

Omelet with any leftover veggies on hand

Snack

Plantain chips

Lunch

Roasted cauliflower soup*◆

Snack

Macadamia nuts with ½ apple

Dinner

Mango shrimp kebobs*

Day 13

Breakfast

Two hard-boiled eggs ◆

½ grapefruit (no sugar added, can add dash of stevia)

Snack

Pear with walnuts

Lunch

Coach Fuel™ green smoothie of choice*

Snack

RXBAR® of choice

Dinner

Grilled chicken breast (salt, pepper, garlic)

Steamed broccoli with melted butter

Roasted cauliflower soup*

Day 13

Breakfast
    Coach Fuel-DF™ chocolate smoothie *(see recipe Page 73)*
Snack
    RXBAR® of choice
Lunch
    Zesty lime, shrimp, and avocado Salad*
Snack
    Macadamia nuts with berries
Dinner
    Low-carb BLT wraps*

Day 14

Breakfast
    Scrambled eggs
    Raw veggie of choice
    Ham
Snack
    Apple
Lunch
    Creamy sweet potato and rosemary soup*◆
Snack
    Almonds
Dinner
    Sautéed salmon in garlic and dill seasoned butter
    Cauliflower rice*

Day 15

Breakfast
    Coach Fuel™ green smoothie*
    Snack
    RXBAR® of choice
Lunch
    Any greens and veggies salad with homemade vinaigrette*
Snack
    Pear with 1 oz. dark chocolate (no sugar added)

Dinner
Seared scallops
Sweet potato and rosemary soup* - *leftover from day 14*

Day 16

Breakfast
Omelet with veggies of choice
Snack
Orange
Lunch
Tomato, cucumber and avocado salad*
Snack
RXBAR® of choice
Dinner
Two small or one large, twice-baked breakfast sweet potatoes*

Day 17

Breakfast
Coach Fuel-DF™ chocolate smoothie *(see recipe page 73)*
Snack
Almonds
Lunch
Sweet potato, bacon and apple hash*
Snack
RXBAR® of choice
Dinner
Burger in lettuce wrap (grass-fed beef preferred, top with homemade mayo,*◆ tomato, avocado, onion, cucumber, pepper, etc.)
Pickles
Raw veggies of choice

Day 18

Breakfast
The pleasures of breakfast salad*
Snack
Raw carrots with paleo ranch dressing*◆

Lunch
> Sautéed veggies (carrots, broccoli, zucchini, cauliflower) with roasted sliced turkey breast

Snack
> Macadamia nuts

Dinner
> Grilled chicken (salt, pepper, garlic)
> Sweet potato oven fries with chipotle mayo*

Day 19

Breakfast
> Coach Fuel™ green smoothie of choice*

Snack
> Raw celery with paleo ranch dressing*◆

Lunch
> Creamy carrot soup*◆

Snack
> RXBAR® of choice

Dinner
> Chicken thighs with root vegetable hash*

Day 20

Breakfast
> Eggs over easy
> Sliced avocado & salt

Snack
> Walnuts with berries

Lunch
> Chicken thighs with veggie hash* - *leftover from day 19*

Snack
> Plantain chips

Dinner
> Ham steak with side of creamy carrot soup* - *leftover from day 19*

Day 21

Breakfast
> Coach Fuel-DF™ chocolate smoothie* *(see recipe page 73)*

Snack

    Apple with almond butter

Lunch

    Green salad with veggies of choice and paleo ranch dressing*◆

Snack

    Guacamole*◆ with raw veggies to dip

Dinner

    Carne Asada* and guacamole*

Day 22

Breakfast

    Zucchini & sweet potato latke's*◆

    Poached egg*

Snack

    Zucchini chips*◆

Lunch

    Coach's pumpkin pie smoothie*

Snack

    RXBAR® of choice

Dinner

    Chicken and zucchini poppers*

    Guacamole to dip*

    Zucchini chips*

Day 23

Breakfast

    Coach Fuel™ green smoothie of choice*

Snack

    Almonds

Lunch

    Mini frittatas*◆

    Berries

Snack

    Apple nachos*

Dinner

    Grilled chicken breast (salt/pepper/garlic)

    Almond roasted heirloom tomatoes*

Day 24

Breakfast

Eggs your choice with uncured organic bacon

Snack

Rosemary and sea salt sweet potato chips*◆

Lunch

Grilled shrimp over greens of choice with homemade vinaigrette*

Snack

Coach's Cocommune™ Bar

Dinner

Grilled or broiled steak of your choice (seasoned to taste)
Roasted cauliflower*

Day 25

Breakfast

Mini frittatas* *(made on Day 23)*
Small green/veggie salad and vinaigrette

Snack

Macadamia nuts

Lunch

Strawberry, cucumber & melon salad*

Snack

Plantain chips (Trader Joe's)

Dinner

Sautéed shrimp (olive oil, garlic, salt, pepper, lemon juice)
Melon slices
Steamed broccoli

Day 26

Breakfast

Coach Fuel-DF™ chocolate smoothie *(see recipe page 73)*

Snack

Raw carrots or cucumbers

Lunch

Tomato, cucumber, and avocado salad*

Snack

    Olives

Dinner

    Oven pork chop pan roast*

    Squash

Day 27

Breakfast

    Eggs your choice with side of uncured bacon

Snack

    Coach's Coconut Almond-DF™ Bar

Lunch

    Lettuce wrap with roast turkey breast meat, avocado, tomato, paleo ranch dressing*

Snack

    Raw celery with almond butter filling

Dinner

    Lip-smackingly good drumsticks*

    Mashed sweet potato

    Small side salad of choice

Day 28

Breakfast

    Coach Fuel™ green smoothie of choice*

Snack

    1 oz. dark chocolate (no added sugar)

    Berries

Lunch

    Omelet with roasted turkey breast meat and veggies of choice

Snack

    Hard-boiled egg ◆

Dinner

    Roast turkey breast, steamed carrots and broccoli, unsweetened applesauce

Day 29

Breakfast

    Two hard-boiled eggs ◆

Snack

    RXBAR® of choice

Lunch

    Creamy chicken, tomato and vegetable soup* (using coconut milk)

Snack

    Pickles

Dinner

    Grilled salmon with avocado salsa*

Day 30

Breakfast

    Coach Fuel-DF™ chocolate smoothie *(see recipe page 73)*

Snack

    Olives

Lunch

    Creamy chicken, tomato and vegetable soup* - *leftover from day 29*

Snack

    Apple with almond butter

Dinner

    Sirloin and peppery tomato reduction*
    Sautéed zucchini & onion

RECIPES

Coach Fuel-DF™ Chocolate Smoothie (can use Coach Fuel™ whey protein if not on the 30-Day Metabolic Comeback Challenge™)

1 scoop Coach Fuel-DF™
8 oz. unsweetened almond, cashew or coconut milk
Dash of cinnamon powder
1 Tbsp. unsweetened cocoa or raw cacao powder
½ banana
½ - 1 tsp. coconut oil
Crushed ice

Fill your blender with all ingredients and blend until desired consistency.   (Add water to thin; use frozen banana to thicken.) Options: Add berries; add a Tbsp. of nut butter; skip cocoa or cacao powder.

Exercise Coach Salsa – simple but delicious!

1 can organic diced tomato
1 can Rotelle brand tomatoes (mild or spicy)
1 handful of cilantro (or 1 tbsp. dried)
1 tsp. garlic powder
1tsp. cumin
1-2 tsp. salt to taste
½ medium onion chopped
1 lime, juiced
1 Jalapeno pepper, seeded and chopped – (optional) for heat

Place ingredients in blender and blend until all are incorporated or to your desired consistency.

Coach's Lettuce Wrap Tacos

Romaine (large leaf) or iceberg lettuce
1 lb. ground beef or turkey (organic; grass fed preferred)
1 medium onion
1 Tbsp. olive oil
1 Tbsp. anchor chili powder
1 tsp. cumin
1 tsp. garlic
1 tsp. dried cilantro
1 tsp. paprika
1 Tbsp. salt
¼ cup water

Optional: chopped tomato, chopped fresh cilantro, chopped avocado

Heat olive oil in pan at medium temperature. Add chopped onion and sauté for two minutes. Add ground beef or turkey. Brown the meat and onion together. Mix the seasonings together and add to the browned meat/onion mixture. Add ¼ cup water. Cook on low for ten minutes.

While meat mixture is cooking, prepare lettuce leaves to use as taco shells. Assemble: add meat, chopped tomato, guacamole and salsa.

TheExerciseCoach.

VEGETARIAN ADDENDUM

The Exercise Coach® Nutrition Playbook™ focuses on eating real, whole food. We strive to help people focus eating vegetables, good sources of protein, fruits, nuts, seeds and other good fats.

The Exercise Coach® Nutrition Playbook™ applies to vegetarians in all areas except for good protein sources. While we believe the best complete sources are found in organic, pastured, grass-fed, animal protein, we realize that this is not a source that vegetarians will select. Protein can be found in plant sources, and eating a diverse array of legumes, some grains, nuts and seeds can give you adequate protein. While information in the Playbook about grains, legumes and soy still applies to vegetarians, we understand you may have more of these food groups in your Eat Daily or Eat Often lists. Our goal is to provide information so that you can make the best choices for yourself.

Some vegetarians incorporate eggs, fish and other seafood into their diets. If this is how you eat, then you are in luck! You can make your protein choices predominantly from these two categories, especially during the 30-Day Metabolic Comeback Challenge,™ where we attempt to eliminate sources of food that contribute to inflammation, insulin spikes, and common food sensitivities.

If you are vegan, then you will simply incorporate the best sources of plant-based proteins (legumes and grains, nuts and seeds). If you usually eat soy, the 30-Day Metabolic Comeback Challenge™ is a good opportunity to eliminate soy and see how your body responds. Soy is very controversial since it has inflammatory properties and is best avoided. If you do plan to eat soy, the best choices are fermented varieties such as tempeh, miso, natto and fermented tofu.

Many vegans/vegetarians do not eat dairy. This is not an issue during the 30-Day Metabolic Comeback Challenge™ or with The Exercise Coach® Nutrition Playbook™. We still recommend you eliminate dairy during the 30-Day Metabolic Comeback Challenge,™ and if you would like to incorporate it into your diet afterward, test by eating for a day and let your body respond for three or four days, and repeat. It is not recommended that you get your main protein sources from dairy for the reasons outlined in The Exercise Coach® Nutrition Playbook™.

The Exercise Coach's® Coach Fuel-DF™ is a great dairy-free vegetarian protein source. While we prefer you get most of your dietary requirements from food sources, Coach Fuel-DF™ is an excellent protein supplement combined with beneficial enzymes, vitamins, and minerals. Make a smoothie for breakfast with your favorite beverage (water, almond milk or coconut milk). Add a dash of unsweetened coco powder, raw cacao powder, coconut oil, cinnamon, veggies, or fresh fruit for variety.

Remember, by following The Exercise Coach® Nutrition Playbook™ you will achieve great benefits by cutting out a significant amount of grains, sugars, artificial sweeteners, junk-food, trans-fats, processed foods, fake foods, dairy, and other bad fats. And, hopefully, you will be incorporating plenty of water into your daily routine for cell nourishment and organ cleansing.

TheExerciseCoach.

MEAL PLANNING FOR THE 30 DAY METABOLIC COMEBACK™

BREAKFAST

Green Veggie/Fruit Smoothie (no added sugars)
Eggs any style (cooked in organic butter or good oil source)
Protein Shake (we suggest Coach Fuel-Dairy Free® for excellent ingredients)

_____

_____

LUNCH

Any breakfast item can be eaten for lunch
Salad w/protein source, with home-made olive oil and vinaigrette style dressing

_____

_____

_____

_____

SNACKS

Nuts	Fruit	Hard boiled eggs
Seeds	raw veggies	_____
Fruit	Nut butters	_____
RXBAR	Plantain Chips	_____
Coach Bar™ (any flavor)	Kale Chips (homemade)	_____

DINNER

Protein / Fat   Vegetables   Fruit

Example:
Chicken / Avocado   Broccoli   Sliced Apples

_____   _____   _____

_____   _____   _____

_____   _____   _____

_____   _____   _____

_____   _____   _____

_____   _____   _____

_____   _____   _____

_____   _____   _____

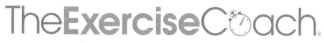

TheExerciseCoach.
Food Journal

Week of_____

Key
P = Protein
C = Carbohydrate
F = Fat

Monday

Breakfast _____   _____

Lunch _____   _____

Dinner _____   _____

_____   _____

Snacks _____   _____

Notes:

Tuesday

Breakfast _____   _____

Lunch _____   _____

Dinner _____   _____

_____   _____

Snacks _____   _____

Notes:

Wednesday

Breakfast _____   _____

Lunch _____   _____

Dinner _____   _____

_____   _____

Snacks _____   _____

Notes:

The Exercise Coach® does not *require* you to keep a food journal. However, we highly *recommend* that you do in order to track the types of foods you are eating, how you feel eating them, and to keep you on track for success! Your Exercise Coach® personal trainer will also be able to give you better guidance based upon actual recorded information. It is recommended you keep all sheets, in order, in a binder and bring at the conclusion of your 30 Day Metabolic Comeback™ as well as at other intervals you discuss.

Thursday

Breakfast _____ _____

Lunch _____ _____

Dinner _____ _____

_____ _____

Snacks _____ _____

Notes:

Friday

Breakfast _____ _____

Lunch _____ _____

Dinner _____ _____

_____ _____

Snacks _____ _____

Notes:

Saturday

Breakfast _____ _____

Lunch _____ _____

Dinner _____ _____

_____ _____

Snacks _____ _____

Notes:

Sunday

Breakfast _____ _____

Lunch _____ _____

Dinner _____ _____

_____ _____

Snacks _____ _____

Notes:

30 DAY CHALLENGE
METABOLICOMEBACK
TESTIMONIALS

Colleen I. – Lake Zurich

I started at The Exercise Coach at the end of January, 2015, as a part of my New Year's resolution to get healthy, lose some weight, and gain more energy. My husband was very supportive and bought me a gift certificate. I did not know anything about The Exercise Coach's workouts or philosophy. The two, 20-minute workouts each week seemed too good to be true. I was also introduced to the February 30 Day Metabolic Comeback Challenge where you eat whole foods, healthy fats, and eliminate gluten, dairy and added sugars. It sounded like the perfect compliment to my new exercise plan. I started to feel better right away! No more bloating after I ate, I had more energy, and the weight started coming off. It was easy to schedule the workouts even with traveling, work, and family commitments. At the end of the 30 days, I couldn't believe I WON the 30 Day Metabolic Comeback Challenge. The formula of nutritious foods and strength exercises really paid off. I highly recommend The Exercise Coach to anyone who wants to feel better, lose weight, and get stronger. It is the easiest program to fit into your life, especially if you work, have children, and have a hectic schedule. The trainers are all friendly, knowledgeable, and are there to support you.

Jerry B. – Fox River Grove

The Exercise Coach has been a blessing in my life. I did the 30 day challenge and I feel really great! I have seen changes in my body, including weight loss and muscle tone, and my wife has also noticed! The 30 day challenge has helped me to change my eating habits and I actually crave healthy foods now. My body is stronger, I have more confidence, and I really enjoy the workouts!

Sue S. – Buffalo Grove

I just finished the 30 Day Challenge! I can hardly believe I am now drinking green smoothies with veggies, almond milk, fruit, and Coach Fuel protein powder. (That is some feat since I never drank shakes due to the texture). As my trainer Mike reminded me, "mind over matter!" Mike was very supportive throughout and always pushed me to push myself, even beyond when I think I can push no more. Stella, the office manager, gave me great tips on the smoothies too! Hopefully I can continue to eat better and continue on the journey.

Candace B. – Scottsdale

I was very pleased with my results. I lost about 9.5 lbs doing the 30 day Metabolic Comeback Challenge and never had any problems sticking to the whole foods plan - I'd even say I enjoyed it. Several things that I focused on were my portion sizes, properly spaced meals and snack times, as well as drinking more water. Also, I have found that I feel so much better, with more energy, and my mood has improved. I plan to stay with the whole foods regimen for the most part. I realize now that strength training AND healthy eating is the cure to reducing FAT!! Thanks to all of the wonderful coaches. I've never ever been a real exerciser and I must say that I enjoy coming to the studio and working out with them! Their encouragement and expertise are greatly appreciated.

Aaron G. – Buffalo Grove

Over the last 30 days I participated in the 30 Day Metabolic Comeback Challenge. To my surprise, I stuck with it 100% and as a result, lost 17 pounds! I feel great and all of my friends and family have taken notice. I totally recommend The Exercise Coach to everyone! Thank you.

Susan M. – Lake Zurich

Over the last 3 years, I've been actively working to improve my health. I've tried many new and old activities that I love such as swimming, kayaking, and walking. I've become more aware of the impact of my food choices and portion sizes. My track record and trajectory over these 3 years has been good and in line with achieving my health and fitness goals. Strength training was missing from my routine. I was surprisingly intimidated by the weights and machines as I had never done this before. A friend recommended The Exercise Coach. So, nine months ago, I put my brave face on, walked in, and signed up. I'm so glad I did. The staff was, and continues to be, very knowledgeable, accepting, and encouraging. I saw results quickly. I'm feeling stronger each month.

After many family celebrations in the fall followed by the holidays, I needed to right my course. I had three months of a less than stellar diet and many hard fought pounds had found their way back to me. I signed up for the Metabolic Comeback Challenge. Again, it was just what I needed. While I've heard some people may have challenges adjusting to changes like this, I thrived on it. I had tons of energy, wasn't hungry, and had no cravings throughout the challenge. The weight I had put on melted away quickly. After 30 days, I'm back to my healthy lifestyle and feeling stronger. I plan to continue a whole-foods based way of eating and checking in at The Exercise Coach twice a week as I work towards my bigger goal of being fit and fabulous by 55!

Cheryl G. – St. Louis

When I began working out at The Exercise Coach, my goals were to improve my overall strength, with emphasis on my core and posture. I was already taking 90-minute hot yoga classes three times a week, so the efficiency of a 20-minute workout was very appealing.

The result from consistently attending my twice-weekly workouts has been an increase in total body muscle strength of 29%. The staff at the Town & Country studio provides me ongoing motivation and also teaches me the science behind the various exercises. Both of these are key to my continual commitment to The Exercise Coach program.

I recently participated in the 30 day Metabolic Comeback Challenge. The staff encouraged me to participate, and provided the knowledge and encouragement for me to succeed. Weight loss was never a prevalent goal, as I was at a relatively healthy weight. The main thing I wanted to gain from the Metabolic Comeback was a reset on some of my eating habits (too much sugar) and also to see if eating whole foods would result in better sleep. Happily, the challenge delivered substantial results: improved sleep, better overall energy & digestive health, and a 14 lb weight loss. During the 30 days I found myself actually enjoying cooking again, and I am looking forward to trying more recipes from the resources at The Exercise Coach. I am thankful to have the staff of Don, Justin, Jessica, Shannon, Jose, and Marissa in my fitness corner, cheering me on.

Barbara C. – Scottsdale

What a wonderful program! I have tried so many weight loss programs (Weight Watchers, LA Weight Loss, etc.) and none compare to The Exercise Coach.

I have always eaten good food and watched my portions, but I still drank my soda and when my energy was down, I would eat a candy bar (usually every day). At the gym, I said "forget it" to personal training. They were more interested in working with the young cute gals. Then, I saw Amanda Coe on Good Morning Arizona – 20 minutes, twice a week! Now this was a program for me! And what a program it is. I started the exercise program in November, 2013, and my stamina after each workout lasts for several days. I went cold turkey on the 30 Day Metabolic Comeback nutrition program and switched from my sodas and candy bars for energy to fruit. It was really easy. I couldn't believe that I didn't miss my root beer.

The plan was so easy. Since my first measurements, I lost 10 inches overall. I am so excited with the results. I am not expecting fast results because it took me a long time to get to the weight I am. By this time next year, I will see some great results and hopefully be very close to my goal. I love flexing my arms and watching that bump jump! My grandkids get a kick out of it! It used to be nothing but flab and now I can actually feel muscle in there. Thank you Amanda Coe and The Exercise Coach! And thank you to the personal trainers that care about the people they are helping. Love you guys!!!

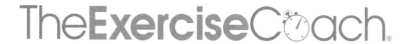

AFTER THE 30-DAY METABOLIC COMEBACK™

FOOD REINTRODUCTION JOURNAL

Date: _____
Name of Food:

_____

Observations: _____

_____

_____

_____

Date: _____
Name of Food:

_____

Observations: _____

_____

_____

_____

Date: _____
Name of Food:

_____

Observations: _____

_____

_____

_____

Date: _____
Name of Food:

_____

Observations: _____

_____

_____

_____

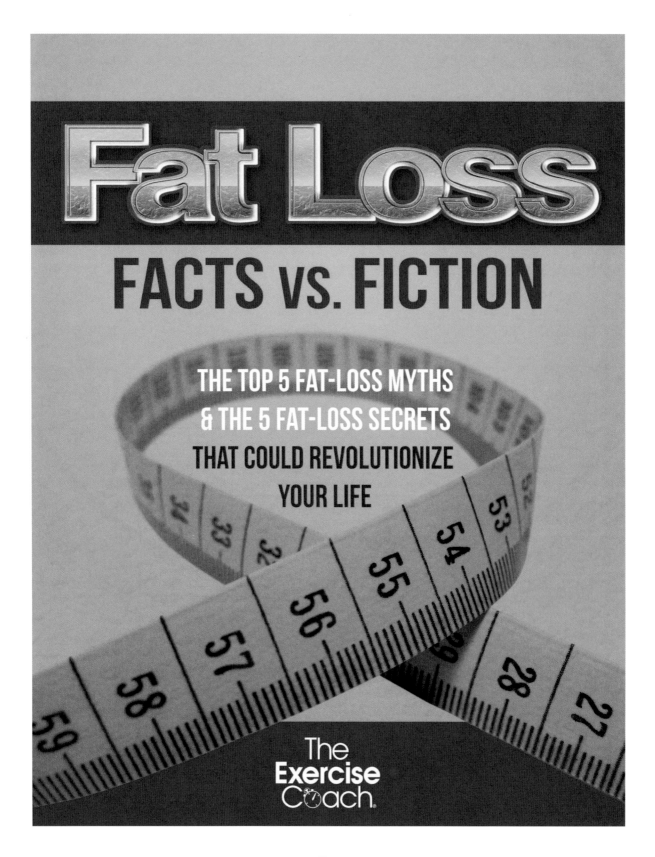

Fat Loss

FACTS vs. FICTION

THE TOP 5 FAT-LOSS MYTHS
& THE 5 FAT-LOSS SECRETS
THAT COULD REVOLUTIONIZE
YOUR LIFE

The
Exercise
Coach.

By
Brian Cygan, CEO, The Exercise Coach®

With type 2 diabetes, heart disease, and America's waistline bulging to frightening highs, it is clear that what we think we know, and what we've been led to believe about fat loss, is not only wrong, but completely backwards. That's right. Your difficulty losing weight is truly not your fault. You have been misinformed for years about healthy eating (i.e., fat makes you fat—replace fat with carbs). You have been misinformed about exercise's role in reducing body fat. And, you have been bombarded by celebrity messages that claim, "This worked for me, so, it will work for you."

At The Exercise Coach® we make it our policy not to cave in to popular fitness trends, but rather to go wherever the science of fat loss and exercise leads us. It is my hope that you take the time to read, understand, and pass along this information to as many people as you can. Share it with others so together you can maximize your fitness and fat-loss efforts while enjoying total freedom from time-consuming and defeating conventional approaches. You can enjoy maximum fitness and fat loss results with just 20-40 minutes of exercise per week—and I will tell you how. First, let's start tearing down the myths. Enjoy!

MYTH #1—AEROBIC EXERCISE IS CRUCIAL FOR FAT LOSS

Everybody's favorite!!! Hop on a treadmill, stepper, elliptical; go for a run, walk, or skip and burn the fat right off. Everyone from the government, to exercise centers, to Nike will have you believe this is the way to go. Unfortunately, research and science do not back this up. Seems simple enough though:

> We eat calories.
> Too many calories make us fat.
> Cardio burns calories.
> Therefore, we become less fat.

Actually, the first 3 statements are all basically true. So what gives? Well first off, cardio burns nowhere near the number of calories we hope it burns. The numbers displayed on exercise equipment are grossly inflated, plus they include your basal metabolic rate (the number of calories your body burns at rest during this time). Another problem is the time it takes to actually burn off one pound of fat. For example, the average 150-pound person burns roughly 100 calories for each mile they run. There are 3,500 calories in one pound of fat, which means you must cover 35 miles to burn the equivalent of one pound of fat. Unfortunately it's not quite that simple, especially when we consider the fact that aerobic activity has been shown to stimulate appetite; and people tend to eat more after exercising.

Another unfortunate side effect of cardio is the increased risk of injury. Take our 150-pound person as an example. If he goes out and runs one mile, he subjects his ankles, hips, knees, and back to over 100 TONS of force. So it becomes a matter of when, not if, he will hurt his back, tear some cartilage in his knee, develop shin splints, or suffer from one of the other numerous injuries that are common to cardio enthusiasts.

Lastly, and arguably the most detrimental consequence of cardio, is that it can actually cause muscle loss over time. This is because during repetitive cardio, you never actually tap into the fibers in your muscles known as fast-twitch muscle fibers. These are the largest, most powerful calorie- (and carbohydrate-) consuming cells in your body. By not utilizing these muscle cells, they atrophy, or waste away. As a side note, fast-twitch doesn't mean fast moving; it means fast to fatigue. That's why these fibers aren't utilized in aerobic exercise. The body uses slow-to-fatigue fibers instead. Fast-twitch fibers are recruited when your body is asked to work against a significant resistance. And the body doesn't see conventional cardio (i.e., walking, jogging, elliptical) as a source of significant resistance.

So look on the bright side, if your goal is fat loss, and you don't like doing cardio (and you're performing safe, effective, and efficient strength-training—more on this later), you can stop doing it. Even if you enjoy these activities, it is important to understand the processes taking place within your body and the inherent dangers associated with the accumulation of force on your joints, muscles, and connective tissue. There is a safer, more concentrated cardio that you can benefit from—but that's a whole different report!

MYTH #2—CALORIC RESTRICTION + WILLPOWER = WEIGHT CONTROL

Everybody knows that if you just eat less, you'll lose fat. Right? WRONG!!! Yes it is true that a caloric deficit must be created within your body to lose weight, however, this alone does NOT guarantee fat loss. Fat loss requires the regulation and control of insulin. Insulin is a hormone. Hormones are like biological instant messages. When they hit a cell membrane, they communicate a specific message to that cell, and the cell reacts. When insulin hits the membrane of a fat cell, it says, "more fatty acids are on the way; make room." And, fat cells are very accommodating to insulin*. In fact, it appears that there is no limit to their ability to make room to store fatty acids. Unfortunately, this means fat cells have an almost limitless ability to grow in size.

So starve the fat cells, right? Well, the problem with caloric restriction is that it puts your body into a catabolic state. Just because you start consuming fewer calories, that doesn't ensure the weight loss comes strictly from your fat. Sure, you will lose *some* fat, but it is estimated 25-50% of the weight one loses from dieting, without strength training, comes from lean mass, i.e., muscle, bone, organs, etc. This means that you will lose muscle, the most metabolically active tissue (calorie-burning tissue) within the body. In addition, calorie restriction can send threat signals throughout your body, causing it to pull some other nifty metabolic tricks to burn fewer calories as a survival technique. This is called adaptive thermogenesis.

These consequences of calorie cutting mean that a return to "normal" eating will even more readily lead to fat accumulation. Did you know that literally 95% of people who "succeed" on a diet regain all the weight they've lost within one year? That's not even the whole story. The majority of people, due to diet-induced muscle loss, end up with even more body fat than before they dieted. This is the danger of what has long been called *yo-yo dieting.* We need to stop talking about "weight-loss" and start talking about "weight-control" strategies. Just look at Oprah's history. Nutrition and exercise strategies must be focused primarily on the creation of sustainable weight loss and the long-term maintenance of muscle.

Additional Information about excess insulin's effect: Food is comprised of 3 macronutrients: carbohydrate and protein (both 4 calories per gram) and fat (9 calories per gram). When we eat protein (necessary for muscular and tissue growth and repair) and fat (promotes healthy cell function), not only does it signal our brains to "stop eating; I'm full," but it has very little—if any—effect on insulin. Carbohydrates (all breads, pastas, grains, chips, junk food, regular soda, cookies, candy, etc.), on the other hand, are converted into sugar, i.e., glucose. Glucose is food for the brain and fuel for our muscles. So after digestion, glucose is absorbed into the blood stream and is used by the brain, our muscles, or is synthesized into glycogen to be stored in the muscles for later use. Unfortunately, our muscles/liver can only store so much glucose, which begs the question—what happens to the extra glucose? The answer is that insulin is called into action to get rid of it. Since insulin has already tried to stuff the excess glucose into our muscles (as glycogen) with no avail, it heads to the liver, which converts it into triglycerides so it can be stored as fat. (*Note*: Elevated triglycerides are a good indicator of serum insulin levels that are too high and are a major risk factor for heart disease and diabetes). Thus, the dangers of excessive carbohydrate consumption cannot only lead to difficulty losing fat, but also put your health at risk. In addition to elevated triglycerides, excess insulin activates an enzyme, which turns the omega-6 fatty acids—so prevalent in the American diet—into a substance called Arachidonic acid. This fatty acid is the building block of a type of hormone that causes inflammation in the body. And, science is demonstrating that inflammation is the root cause of heart disease, stroke, some cancers, autoimmune deficiencies, and brain disorders.

MYTH #3—"CORE" EXERCISES ARE TUMMY TONERS

When I look at this one I think, "C'mon, nobody really believes that." However, my experience working with thousands of people confirms it has a firm hold on its position as one of the most propagated fat-loss myths. Over the holidays, I read an article featured on a popular Internet news site that read:

"Achieving a toned, sexy tummy might seem like a pipe dream this time of year. Baggy sweaters abound, eggnog is served, and Frosty the Snowman doesn't offer much in the way of flat-belly inspiration. But getting a <u>sleek, sexy stomach</u> is easier than you think. Spend just five minutes a day on toning your abs and you'll get an amazing middle."

WRONG! Today people refer to strengthening exercises for the mid-section as "core" exercises. Now, there is a lot of confusion surrounding the term "core," but before I get to that, I'd like to focus on the word "toning." Look at that excerpt again. It says a "toned" tummy can be achieved by "toning" exercises. This is simply *not* true.

The term *tone*, scientifically speaking, refers to the residual tension in a muscle at rest. And, by strengthening a muscle, you do tend to improve its tone or make it firmer. However, this is not what the writer above—or most people for that matter—mean when they use the term tone or toning. Instead, they believe that performing exercises for the muscles in a specific area of the body makes that area leaner. So, they believe that exercising the abdominals will flatten their tummy. Exercise scientists have described this myth as the spot-reduction myth. It's biologically impossible. Strengthening the *muscles* in your mid-section has no impact on the *fat* that lies on top of them. Your fat cells don't even know that you are exercising.

Imagine if this myth were reality. You could literally exercise the fat off of one side of your body. But, we know intuitively and from science that it doesn't work that way. Researchers once looked at the dominant arm of pro tennis players to see if it was leaner than their non-dominant arm. The results: While it was a little more muscular, it was not less fat. This demonstrates that when fat cells are tapped by your body for energy, they are accessed from all over, not just from the area being exercised.

Your body actually has a preference for the order in which it will burn fat from your body. Unfortunately for all of us, the fat cells on the stomach come off last. You can do crunches until you can't move, but you will lose fat from your arms, legs, and earlobes before your body decides to take it from the midsection. Unfortunately, you can't change your body's mind on this one. That tummy can be flattened though. You just have to work your way through the fat cells in the rest of your body before you get there.

MYTH #4—STRENGTH TRAINING CAUSES BULKINESS

Weight loss has a powerful impact on a person's wellness. Equally motivating for most people, though, are their appearance-based goals. Women want to fit into their skinny jeans or go sleeveless. Men want to rid themselves of the all too common spare tire. In simple terms, people want to be smaller, not larger. I've found that for many people, this creates an understandable, yet unwarranted, and counter-productive fear of building muscle.

I can't count the number of times I've told someone the number one goal of exercise should be to build muscle only to hear, "No, No. I don't want to build muscle. I want to lose weight."

What the client means is, "I am afraid that building muscle will make me bigger than I already feel." But, building muscle is absolutely critical for maximizing fat loss results, so we need to deal with this myth.

First of all, most people do not have the ability to build large muscles. The potential for increases in muscle size is determined primarily by two things: geometry and genetic expression.

GEOMETRY

On the flip side of the "bulky" myth is the myth that any guy that wants large muscles can do so by following a "bodybuilding" type program. I've had to gently squash the aspirations of many young men looking to get "huge." Based on my experience and understanding of anatomy, I can usually tell within seconds of looking at someone if they have the capacity to be the next Arnold Schwarzenegger or not. To make it more concrete, I point out the following: A muscle's capacity to grow in thickness is based on the ratio between the length of the actual muscle versus the visible length of that muscle tendon. Let me give you an example. Bend your arm to 90 degrees at the elbow. Now measure the number of finger widths you can fit between your bicep and forearm. If the answer is two or more, don't worry—Arnold you are not!

GENES

The other major determinant of muscle size has to do with the expression of the gene known as myostatin. Research has been done on individuals with abnormally large muscles and, by and large, their myostatin expression is very limited. Fortunately, most of us have myostatin that is speaking loud and clear to the body saying, "Hey, get stronger, but don't get bigger. It costs too much metabolically." Probably less than one person out of every hundred-thousand possesses myostatin that allows the building of very large muscles.

One final consideration is the actual amount of space fat tissue takes up compared to muscle. Remember that the average person loses about five pounds of muscle per decade after age thirty. So the average forty-year-old had a little more muscle, not less, ten years prior when they were happier with their figure (physique for you guys reading this).

It's hard work to put back on those five pounds. Most people are lucky to do that. Any more than that would be rare. Now consider that fat takes up a lot more space than muscle. Five pounds of fat is about as voluminous as a gallon milk jug. Now picture five pounds of ground round. It doesn't take up nearly as much space. So if you gain five pounds of muscle and lose five pounds of fat, guess what? You are smaller. And, most people at age forty have more than five pounds of fat to lose.

So practically every forty-year-old in America has a greater potential to get smaller through fat loss than they do to grow larger through muscle building. Do not fear muscle. It's your best fat-loss friend.

MYTH #5—I'VE TRIED EVERYTHING!

Most of the people we meet at The Exercise Coach® obviously don't believe this one. They realize they haven't tried our cutting-edge approach. So, this one is for you people out there who need to be moved from contemplating change to taking action.

Maybe you have tried dieting techniques from low-carb to low-fat and everything in between. You've done cardio, crunches, and core conditioning. All you have to show for it is the bill and some time lost. I understand how the plethora of misinformation circulating in textbooks, exercise books, health clubs, and around the water cooler can make you *feel* like you have tried everything.

The good news is you can discover the truth for yourself at The Exercise Coach® where we maximize your fitness and fat loss with just two, 20-minute workouts per week. Come in and meet with one of our friendly, expert instructors. Until then, let me give you a brief explanation of some key components of The Exercise Coach® approach.

SECRET #1—EATING FOR IMPACT

The Exercise Coach® specializes in cutting-edge exercise concepts. It's our passion. So we know very well what exercise can do and what exercise cannot do. We know that exercise is vital for optimal fat-loss results. However, we are well aware, and you need to be too, that when it comes to weight loss, the formula is exercise + Proper nutrition = healthy weight loss. More specifically, whole-effort exercise + whole-food nutrition = a whole new you.

It's to this end that we constantly educate our clients and empower them with convenient nutrition solutions. Our aim is to help our clients understand that food no longer has to be the enemy. In fact, food can become your greatest wellness and weight-control ally.

Everything you eat has a powerful effect on your physiology. You just need to understand the effect that various foods have. Once you do, you can eat <u>for</u> the positive contribution to your efforts that food can make instead of <u>despite</u> the negative impact.

Nutrition can be confusing and intimidating, so we like to narrow down your focus to four areas that will give you the biggest bang for your buck of effort. I'll give you a brief summary here to get you thinking about how you are doing in these areas.

Hunger Control: Make no mistake about it. You cannot eat an excess of calories or carbohydrates and expect to lose weight. However, I think that biology has a lot more to do with your ability to stay the course than will power does. There are several strategies available to help you achieve an outstanding degree of satiety from your meals. Maybe the single most important is consuming adequate (not excessive) amounts of protein at the right time throughout the day. Start by looking at your breakfast. Most people don't eat protein for breakfast, but it can have a huge impact on satiety if you do. Remember this: Carbohydrates grow in the ground and proteins are things that move around. Make sure you eat protein as part of your breakfast and at every snack and meal through the day.

Insulin Control: Insulin is a storage signal. It tells your fat cells to go into *buy and hold mode*. The more insulin you have in your bloodstream, the stronger the signal.

The best way to keep insulin under control is to eat the proper kinds and amount of carbohydrates. The easiest way to do this is to stick with fruits and vegetables.

Remember, your muscles and brain need carbohydrates to fuel them. Restricting carbs too much will only backfire on you. It will lead to extreme fatigability and excess levels of cortisol (a stress hormone). This actually makes your body produce excess insulin as well. So the best approach is to stay away from diet plans that include the words *high* or *low*. These tend to be unsustainable. Moderation is the key.

Fatty Acid Control: Fatty acids make up cell membranes and are also the building blocks for a type of hormone known as an eicosanoid. Two very important fatty acids are Omega-6 and Omega-3 fatty acids. Research has shown that people who consume these in appropriate ratios are much healthier and have a better chance of losing fat. This is due to reduced inflammation in the body and more hormonally responsive cells.

Damage Control: From a wellness and longevity point of view, your body is always trying to strike a balance between damage and repair. For most of us, better damage control is what we need. This can be achieved by eating lots of green leafy vegetable and dark-colored berries. Today there are also many good products on the market that provide concentrated amounts of the phytochemicals found in these foods.

SECRET #2—THE MUSCULAR MINDSET

Most everyone thinks we should *exercise,* but few understand what the paramount goal in exercise should be. Undeniably, unequivocally, no question about it—the emphatic answer is to BUILD MUSCLE. Increased muscle mass is the lead domino in a lineup of health and fitness markers. These include metabolism, strength, endurance, bone density, blood pressure, and cholesterol levels. As muscles are conditioned, these other markers improve. When you lose muscle as you age, these markers will follow in suit and worsen. In a recent landmark study, increasing muscle strength was even shown to reverse aging at the level of DNA in a way that literally no other intervention ever has.

When it comes to fat loss, you need to have what we call "The Muscular Mindset." The only way to maximize the loss of body-fat is to make sure any weight you lose comes from fat—not muscle. This is called discriminated weight loss. The only way to do this is to focus on strengthening exercise. In fact, the best results tend to be for those people who do proper strength training only. That's right, *no* conventional cardio. Just my opinion? Nope.

Two renowned researchers combined their findings looking at the effects of diet alone, diet + strength training, and diet + aerobics and strength training. Look at the results.

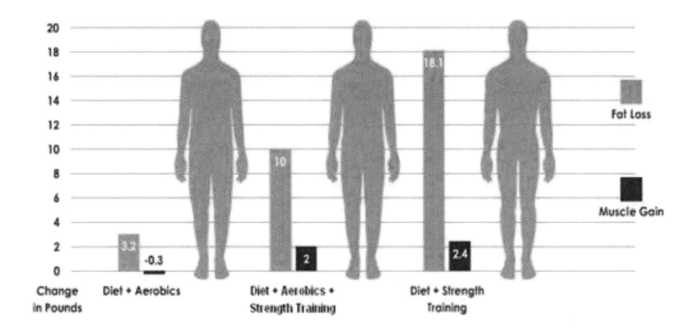

Westcott and Darden found that the most effective fat loss approach was to combine a specific kind of strength training with appropriate nutrition. What's more, they determined that anything beyond the minimum amount of exercise necessary to build muscle was actually counter-productive. In their studies, the strength training-only subjects lost almost *twice* as much fat as those who combined strength training with aerobics.

So what exactly is the secret to making strength training this effective? I'm glad you asked.

SECRET #3—THE HIGH-INTENSITY BREAKTHROUGH

OK. I'll let you in on the secret. The form of strength training used in the Westcott/Darden studies was a type of strength training known as HIT. That stands for High-Intensity Training. Intensity is by far the most important variable to manipulate in an exercise program. What is intensity? It can be defined simply as the degree of momentary effort utilized in an exercise. So we could call the maximum amount of exertion you could call upon at a given moment, 100-percent intensity. Conversely, we could call sitting on the couch a goose egg on the intensity indicator. Walking would be closer to the couch than it would be to your maximum effort.

Now before I go on, let me emphasize that, when we talk about intensity, we are talking about YOUR momentary abilities, not an Olympic athlete's. Well, unless that is whom we are talking about. You see, we have created programs powered by technology that are smart enough to adapt to the unique abilities of all kinds of exercisers. Our average client is about 55 years old, and we work very successfully with younger athletes and men and women well into their 80's. High-intensity does not mean safety is compromised. In fact, the type of work we perform at

The Exercise Coach® is better characterized as "Right-Intensity Training™." So why is intensity so important? Well, your body was designed to be very economical. That is, it will only make changes that it determines are necessary. Changes that are costly and unnecessary won't be made. The synthesis of new muscle tissue is very costly metabolically. And, while we know you need it, your body needs to be convinced. That's what exercise is—the intelligent application of a physiological stressor in order to give your body a reason to change, adapt, or upgrade if you will. When you perform adequately challenging muscular work (i.e., intense), alarms go off in your physiology saying, "Wow! Is that a bear you are fighting with? Are you running from a lion?" And, since there is no bear or lion and you survive the encounter, your body takes all the resources at its disposal and uses them to better prepare you for your next battle (perceived battle, that is).

Now, the really cool part is that when you work hard enough to stimulate your body to adapt, it takes time for the changes to be made. We call that the recovery period. It's vitally important to understand that you aren't getting more fit during exercise, but rather during the rest period after. Most people will require a minimum of 48-72 hours of rest. And, we don't want to exercise before that because it's at best a waste of time and, worst case scenario, it stunts your body's positive response (i.e., diminishes your results). So high-intensity exercise should be performed infrequently. About twice per week is ideal. Just think of what you can do with all the time-savings.

The other cool part is that when you exercise at adequate intensity levels, it requires that you don't work out very long. In fact, you can't. On average, a high-intensity strength workout lasts about 15-20 minutes. Where does that duration come from? Exercise that qualifies as high-intensity challenges your muscles in a manner that couldn't be sustained for more than about 1-2 minutes, even if your life depended on it. And, once you have done a high-intensity strength training set, you have done what you can to set your adaptive machinery in motion. Multiple sets are NOT necessary. Westcott and Darden both subscribe to a "one-set" per muscle group approach as a result of the research we showed you. The key is understanding that it's not just "using" a muscle for 1-2 minutes that triggers results. It's a sufficiently high level of effort that is the stimulus. That's why a professional trainer who is committed to this type of training comes in very handy. We can help you find the load and effort levels that are just right for you. At The Exercise Coach®, we do this in a way that nobody else does. The processes and technologies we utilize give us the ability to measure your unique muscular make up and deliver a strength training stimulus that is as unique to you as your fingerprint. This means fast results!

Relative to fat loss, intensity in exercise moves us beyond worrying about the archaic measure of calories burned during exercise. That's so 1980's.

Cutting edge exercise professionals are more interested in helping you trigger responses that are exclusive to High-Intensity Training. These include, but are not limited to:

Increased Pulsatile HGH: HGH, or Human Growth Hormone, is a hormone that is a powerful fat-burner. It is released at night while sleeping and at intervals throughout the day. Your

HGH releases decrease with age. The best way to increase HGH output is with meaningful exertion. One study showed a 560% increase in HGH after just several minutes of intense exercise.

Increased EPOC: EPOC stands for Excess Post-Exercise Oxygen Consumption. After intense exercise, your body has to expend a lot of energy putting itself back together, metabolically speaking. So, while you may burn fewer total calories _during_ a brief high-intensity exercise session, in the end, you burn more _as a result_ of your efforts. Your energy expenditure increases last up to four days after intense exercise.

Increased Insulin Sensitivity: I've talked about insulin a lot already. Proper strength training can enhance your muscle cells' ability to uptake and utilize glucose (i.e., blood sugar), thereby requiring less insulin production by your body. Less insulin in your blood means weaker fat storage signals, stronger fat mobilization signals, and better health.

Fat-loss research is showing these and other recently discovered exercise effects are the keys to exercising for maximum fat loss. Furthermore, many experts (real experts, that is) believe that it's literally impossible for some people to lose fat in a healthy manner without intense muscular conditioning.

So find someone who can help you with the specifics of effective high-intensity strength training strategies. Just make sure they have a lot of experience with these techniques and understand how to make this form of exercise not only the most effective, but also the safest possible. There is one variable that must be focused on if this is to be the case. Let me share with you the secret to safety in strength training.

SECRET #4—CONTROLLED MUSCULAR LOADING

As I mentioned before, at The Exercise Coach® we work with people ranging in age from 12 up to 80 years plus. Some of our clients are women that come to us for the purpose of preventing and reversing osteoporosis. As you know, osteoporotics have weakened bones, yet the type of exercise we do is so safe, it allows them to work hard enough to stimulate bone density increases. Researchers from Tufts University agree. Their studies indicate that even among 90-year-olds, there is a greater risk associated with _not_ doing intense strength than there is participating in it.

In addition, we've worked with people with a variety of orthopedic challenges and many, many, many people with little to no exercise experience. Maybe the most revolutionary aspect of our program is that, unlike any other, it allows us to simultaneously increase the intensity of exercise and the safety of exercise. How is that possible? That's a good question, because outside of our approach, it can't be done.

Here is the greatest secret, bar none, to maximizing weight-lifting safety—eliminate explosive movement and impact force. Have you ever noticed how most people sort of heave and thrust weights around or move their body in a ballistic manner? This is the fast track to what we call the fitness fallout. Injuries happen when some part of your body is exposed to a force that exceeds its structural integrity. The best way to avoid that is to limit force. This doesn't necessarily mean you lift light weights. They can be just as dangerous. In fact, in many cases they are MORE dangerous than heavier weights because they allow such rapid movement, change in direction, and therefore joint force. It's been reported that emergency rooms around the country are seeing dozens of people per day with joint injuries from "fitness" activities using gaming systems. This is because, with its rapid movements, there are inherently high-forces just like running and ballistic weight-lifting.

For two decades, I've been committed to helping my clients understand that there is literally no reason to perform explosive exercise movements. It only increases the risk of injury. That's why we use controlled movements when we exercise at The Exercise Coach®. Controlled muscle loading reduces joint force, makes it easier to maintain proper form, and affords our clients the confidence they need to work hard enough to make their exercise matter. In fact, with our proprietary connected strength technologies, all of the muscular loading is user-generated and, therefore, individually appropriate. You really need to experience this breakthrough exercise format to appreciate it.

With weights, proper speed of movement varies from exercise to exercise, based on a host of factors (I'll spare you the physics lesson). Just remember, when in doubt—MOVE SLOWER. Broadly speaking, take about 5-10 seconds to raise a weight and about 5-10 seconds to lower it. Even better (shameless plug coming up), work with a company that has helped thousands of people transform their bodies and understands how to perfectly personalize exercise for any individual's needs.

SECRET #5—THE GUIDED EXERCISE ADVANTAGE

Losing fat, changing your lifestyle, and becoming healthier can be an extremely daunting task and something not easily conveyed within 10 concepts. As you probably already know, there is tons of misinformation circulating about and, with jobs and families to tend to, you only have so much time to discover the truth. But that's what we are here for. At The Exercise Coach®, we are passionate about partnering with you to help you reach your goals. According to writer Alan Deutschman, that might be the most valuable aspect of what we do. Deutschman's book, *Change or Die*, asks this question, "Can you change when change matters most?" He found that even those individuals faced with serious threats to their health could not change unless they entered into a helpful relationship with someone who could inject confidence and direction into the situation. Let me tell you something. I am confident that you can achieve lasting weight loss. Despite past attempts that didn't pan out, I know you can do this. It would be our privilege to provide you with the expert guidance and encouraging accountability you need.

For a little inspiration, I'd like to leave you with a few success stories. Check out these success-ful clients of ours! They committed to the principles outlined here and transformed their bodies and lives in ways they could hardly believe. You can do it too!

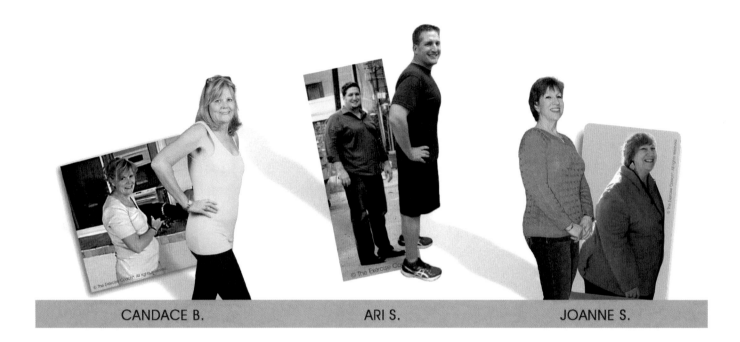

CANDACE B.   ARI S.   JOANNE S.

TheExerciseCoach.

GREAT NON-DAIRY SOURCES OF CALCIUM

Food Source	Amount	mg Calcium/per
Orange Juice w/added calcium	1 cup	350
Sardines	3 oz.	325
Collard Greens	1 cup	300
Mustard Greens	1 cup	276
Pink Salmon, canned w/bone	3 oz.	181
Broccoli	1 med. Stalk	180
Spinach (cooked)	½ cup	146
Turnip Greens (cooked)	½ cup	124
Kale (cooked)	½ cup	90
Blue Crab (canned)	3 oz.	86
Almonds	¼ cup	83
Butternut Squash	1 cup	82
Clams (canned)	3 oz.	78
Orange	1 large	76
Blackberries	1 cup	46
Pineapple Juice	1 cup	42
Almond Milk	Coconut Milk (365 | Trader Joe | So Delicious)		varies per brand

Source: Nutrient values from Agricultural Research Service (ARS) Nutrient Database for Standard Reference, Release 17.

HEALTHY OILS: WHICH TO EAT WHICH TO DITCH

WHICH TO EAT:

HIGH HEAT
(450+ DEGREES)

Avocado Oil (not virgin)
Ghee (clarified butter)
Olive Oil, high-quality, extra light
Palm Oil

MEDIUM-LOW HEAT
(250-324 DEGREES)

Any on the High, Med-High, or
 Medium Heat Lists
Butter, organic
Sesame Seed Oil, unrefined
Walnut oil, unrefined

MEDIUM HIGH HEAT
(375-449 DEGREES)

Any on the High Heat List
Olive Oil, virgin
Almond Oil
Macadamia Nut Oil
Coconut Oil, refined
Tallow (beef)

LOW HEAT
(225-249 DEGREES)

Any on the High, Med-High, Medium
 or Medium-Low Heat Lists
Pistachio Oil

COLD
(BEST TO CHOOSE ORGANIC, COLD PRESSED FORMS)

Olive Oil, extra virgin
Sesame Oil
Nut Oils
Avocado Oil

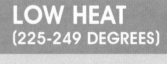

MEDIUM HEAT
(324-374 DEGREES)

Any on the High or Med-High
 Heat Lists
Olive Oil, extra virgin
Lard
Coconut Oil, unrefined

HEALTHY OILS: WHICH TO EAT WHICH TO DITCH

WHICH TO DITCH:

These oils contain trans-fats or are highly processed and oxidize easily with light, air or heat. And, they are not included in our healthy fats list.

Margarine
Hydrogenated or partially hydrogenated oils
Man-made trans-fats often found in "buttery spreads"
   including oil blends like Earth Balance, Benecol and
   I Can't Believe It's Not Butter, to name a few
Canola Oil (also known as rapeseed oil)
Corn Oil
Vegetable Oil
Soybean Oil
Grapeseed Oil
Sunflower Oil
Safflower Oil
Rice Bran Oil

*Healthy oils placed in their "heat" category based on their smoke point
(https://en.wikipedia.org/wiki/Smoke_point)

HEALTHY SNACK IDEAS
— AT WORK OR ON THE GO —

If you're like most people, you make a plan to eat better! Breakfast begins the day just great with a nice green protein shake filled with spinach, protein powder, berries and coconut oil. Lunch is a green salad with organic chicken, kale, chopped egg, veggies, and olive oil with balsamic vinegar dressing. And, dinner will be 5-Star: salmon sautéed with garlic and dill, with a side of steamed carrots. You're feeling really great about your efforts!

Uh oh! Sometime around midafternoon, hunger sets in. You're at work or on the go and you can't run out and find a healthy snack that won't blow your hard work! You know you should have brought something from home, but you were so busy planning your three healthy meals that day, time got away from you.

Here's what you do. Plan ALL your snacks out. Not for just one day, but every day.

Then, every day that you wish to have a healthy snack, you simply eat an allowed snack and your hunger pains won't stand a chance. When you are hungry is the worst time to think of a snack you wish to eat. It's also the worst time to go grocery shopping. You need to always be on offense when it comes to snack time and hunger in-between meals.

There are many healthy snacks to choose from, but remember: having too many to choose from creates more work. Pick from a handful that you actually like, not ones you are settling for just because you believe they are good for you. When you settle, hunger pains can actually still win because you may reject your choice. When you actually like your snack, you will choose to eat it because it's delicious. You probably will look forward to snack time.

Here are some of my favorites. Some contain chocolate!!

Handfuls of nuts, seeds, coconut flakes and dried fruit*
Pick which type you like and prepare small bags or containers with them in advance. Treat yourself by putting in a few dark chocolate pieces. Choose dark chocolate with no added sugars.

Antioxidant dark chocolate bark*
Make a big batch and store in small bags or containers in the fridge. (recipe located on www.exercisecoach. com/resources/nutritional information).

Cacao powder protein shake

If you have a break room at work, keep an individual size smoothie blender on hand and whip one up. Cacao powder, almond or coconut milk, protein powder (Coach Fuel or Coach Fuel-DF recommended), and a little bit of ice. You can also add a dollop of nut butter or various fruits to keep it interesting.

Apples with almond or cashew butter

Chop up an apple in the morning and add a splash of lemon juice to keep from it from browning. Scoop a tablespoon of nut butter into a bowl and dip your apple to enjoy the great-tasting combo. Works well with bananas too!

Guacamole

A batch can last two to three days if sealed properly. Dip fresh veggies like carrots, peppers or celery. (recipe on www.exercisecoach.com/resources/nutritional information).

Raw veggies

Chop ahead and put in snack packs to go! Carrots, celery, peppers, cauliflower, broccoli, mushrooms, cucumbers, etc. Mix and match. Dip in nut butters, guacamole, or homemade vinaigrette dressing (recipe on www.exercisecoach.com/resources/nutritional information).

Fresh fruits

Any individual fruits that you like, or a variety. Chop ahead and put in snack packs. (If you have issues with blood sugar, choose blackberries, raspberries or strawberries, which are lower in sugar).

Plantain chips

Crunchy and sweet ! Trader Joe's has them ready to go!

Avocado

Scoop out half one day and half the next. Seal tightly to keep from browning.

RXBAR®

They come in a variety of flavors and have only five natural ingredients! No added sugars! Rxbar.com or at your local The Exercise Coach® Studio.

Grapes

Have a handful with an ounce or two of raw milk cheese* (sold at Whole Foods or Trader Joe's).

Hard-boiled eggs

Have one or two – they're only about 70 calories each. Tons of nutrition are packed into this easy-to-eat snack. Have some salt or pepper on hand to season. Make a dozen for the week!

Start planning your own snack attack packs, and be ready when between-meal hunger sets in!

*Dried fruit and any form of cheese is not allowed during The 30 Day Metabolic Comeback Challenge.™

Resource and Reference Links

The following resource and reference links may prove helpful to your quest for great nutrition and health. Simply type in the URL into your browser to search. All direct links can also be accessed at www.exercisecoach.com / password: **comeback30days#**

ALCOHOLIC BEVERAGES

- http://www.hsph.harvard.edu/nutritionsource/alcohol-full-story/
- https://www.yahoo.com/news/7-amazing-health-benefits-drinking-red-wine-144532108.html?ref=gs
- http://www.medicinenet.com/alcohol_and_nutrition/page4.htm

ARTIFICIAL SWEETENERS

- http://www.medicinenet.com/artificial_sweeteners/article.htm
- http://www.globalhealingcenter.com/natural-health/two-of-the-most-dangerous-artificial-sweeteners/
- http://www.nutralegacy.com/blog/general-healthcare/top-10-dangers-of-artificial-sweeteners-full/
- http://drhyman.com/blog/2015/12/02/why-you-should-ditch-artificial-sweeteners/
- http://drhersh.blogspot.com/2015/10/is-truvia-same-as-stevia.html

BONE BROTH

- http://eatlocalgrown.com/article/11784-benefits-bone-broth.html

BOOKS ON NUTRITION, HEALTHY LIVING

- Eat Fat, Get Thin, by Mark Hyman, M.D.
- Smart Fat, Steven Masley, M.D. and Jonny Bowden, Ph.D., CNS
- Sugar Shock, Connie Bennett, C.H.H.C., with Stephen Sinatra, M.D.

- <u>150 Healthiest Foods on Earth</u>, by Jonny Bowden, Ph.D., CNS
- <u>150 Healthiest 15 Minute Recipes on Earth,</u> by Jeannette Bessinger and Jonny Bowden, Ph.D., CNS
- <u>Tox-Sick</u>, by Suzanne Somers
- <u>Wheat Belly,</u> by William Davis, M.D.
- <u>The Anti-Inflammation Zone</u>, by Barry Sears, M.D.
- <u>Nature's Safest, Most Effective Anti-Inflammatory – Fish Oil</u>, by Joseph C. Maroon, M.D. and Jeffrey Bost, P.A.C.
- <u>Body by Science</u>, by Doug McGuff, M.D. and John Little
- <u>Why Stomach Acid is Good For You,</u> by Jonathan Wright, M.D. and Lane Lenard, Ph.D.
- <u>No More Heartburn</u>, by Sherry A. Rogers, M.D.

BUTTER

- http://bodyecology.com/articles/benefits_of_real_butter.php
- http://www.westonaprice.org/?s=butter&submit=Search

CANCER

- http://www.ewg.org/cancer/?inlist=Y/utm_source=201605CancerRelease&utm_medium=email&utm_campaign=201605CancerRelease

CARRAGEENAN

- http://wellnessmama.com/2925/what-is-carrageenan/
- http://www.drweil.com/drw/u/QAA401181/ls-Carrageenan-Safe.html
- http://www.prevention.com/food/healthy-eating-tips/carrageenan-natural-ingredient-you-should-ban-your-diet

CHOLESTEROL: DEBUNKING THE MYTHS

- <u>The Cholesterol Hoax</u>, by Sherry A. Rogers, M.D.
- http://www.fitday.com/fitness-articles/nutrition/healthy-eating/food-myths-debunked-eating-eggs-raises-your-cholesterol-level.html
- http://blog.exercisecoach.com/cholesterol-does-not-cause-heart-disease/
- http://blog.exercisecoach.com/high-cholesterol-vs-low-cholesterol/
- http://blog.exercisecoach.com/why-we-need-cholesterol/
- http://blog.exercisecoach.com/the-truth-about-cholesterol-where-did-we-go-wrong/
- https://www.lewrockwell.com/2013/05/joseph-mercola/the-great-cholesterol-scam/

COCONUT WATER

- http://www.bustle.com/articles/43279-9-best-coconut-water-brands-according-to-experts
- http://foodbabe.com/2014/07/15/how-to-buy-the-healthiest-coconut-water-and-avoid-the-worst/

DAIRY

- http://time.com/4279538/the-case-against-low-fat-milk-is-stronger-than-ever/?xid=tcoshare
- http://drhyman.com/blog/2010/06/24/dairy-6-reasons-you-should-avoid-it-at-all-costs-2/
- http://articles.mercola.com/sites/articles/archive/2014/09/29/full-fat-dairy-products.aspx
- http://amazingwellnessmag.com/dairy-fact-and-fiction/
- http://acaai.org/allergies/types-allergies/food-allergy/types-food-allergy/milk-dairy-allergy
- http://time.com/4279538/low-fat-milk-vs-whole-milk/?xid=tcoshare
- http://www.realmilk.com/real-milk-finder/
- IGF-1 (Growth Factor): http://www.veganlifestylecoach.com/Vegan_Lifestyle_Coach/Andys_blog/Entries/2009/4/20_DAIRY-_IGF_-_1_INSULIN-LIKE_GROWTH_FACTOR_1.html
- Allergy Symptoms: http://www.mayoclinic.org/diseases-conditions/milk-allergy/basics/symptoms/con-20032147

DIABETES, INSULIN RESISTANCE, HIGH BLOOD SUGAR

- http://www.diabetes.org/diabetes-basics/statistics/
- http://www.niddk.nih.gov/health-information/health-topics/Diabetes/insulin-resistance-pre-diabetes/Pages/index.aspx
- http://abcnews.go.com/Health/DiabetesOverview/story?id=3843485
- http://www.emedicinehealth.com/high_blood_sugar_hyperglycemia/article_em.htm

EGGS

- http://whfoods.com/genpage.php?tname=foodspice&dbid=92
- https://authoritynutrition.com/6-reasons-why-eggs-are-the-healthiest-food-on-the-planet/

ENVIRONMENTAL TOXICITY

- <u>Tox-Sick</u>, Suzanne Sommers
- www.ewg.org
- http://www.onegreenplanet.org/lifestyle/hidden-toxins-in-our-everyday-lives-and-how-to-avoid-them/

FATS

- <u>Smart Fat</u>, Jonny Bowden, Ph.D., CNS
- <u>Eat Fat, Get Thin</u>, Mark Hyman, M.D.
- http://time.com/4279538/low-fat-milk-vs-whole-milk/?xid=tcoshare
- http://articles.mercola.com/sites/articles/archive/2011/09/01/enjoy-saturated-fats-theyre-good-for-you.aspx
- http://www.marksdailyapple.com/why-eating-animals-makes-everything-easier/
- http://drhyman.com/blog/2016/01/08/why-fat-doesnt-make-you-fat/
- What are Omega 3 Fatty acids? http://umm.edu/health/medical/altmed/supplement/omega3-fatty-acids
- Imbalance of Omega 6 to Omega 3 Fatty Acids: http://www.ncbi.nlm.nih.gov/pubmed/12442909
- Trans Fats: https://authoritynutrition.com/why-trans-fats-are-bad/

FIBER

- http://www.webmd.com/diet/insoluble-soluble-fiber
- http://www.livestrong.com/article/114903-highest-insoluble-fiber-content-foods/
- http://www.doctoroz.com/blog/jodi-sawyer-rn/why-fiber-so-important
- http://www.mayoclinic.org/healthy-lifestyle/nutrition-and-healthy-eating/in-depth/fiber/art-20043983?pg=2

FISH OIL

- The Exercise Coach® Omega Ultra or Omegade (Designs for Health)
- http://www.designsforhealth.com
- https://www.nordicnaturals.com
- http://www.sfh.com/shop/omega-3-oil/

FODMAPS

- <u>The Complete Low Fodmap Diet</u>, by Sue Shepherd, PhD and Peter Gibson, M.D.

FOOD SENSITIVITIES, ALLERGIES

- http://drhyman.com/blog/2012/02/22/how-hidden-food-sensitivities-make-you-fat/
- http://shepherdworks.com.au/disease-information/low-fodmap-diet

GMOS (GENETICALLY MODIFIED ORGANISMS)

- http://www.foodrenegade.com/link-between-roundup-ready-gmos-disease/
- http://responsibletechnology.org/10-reasons-to-avoid-gmos/
- http://www.nongmoproject.org/learn-more/

GRAINS

- Wheat Belly, William Davis, M.D.
- http://paleoleap.com/what-is-wrong-with-grains/
- http://wellnessmama.com/575/problem-with-grains/
- http://www.livestrong.com/article/272384-how-to-follow-a-diet-without-grains-sugar/

GLYCEMIC INDEX (GI) AND LOAD (GL)

- http://www.glycemicindex.com/about.php
- http://nutritiondata.self.com

GLUTEN

- https://authoritynutrition.com/6-shocking-reasons-why-gluten-is-bad/
- http://www.mindbodygreen.com/0-7482/10-signs-youre-gluten-intolerant.html
- http://www.arthritis.org/living-with-arthritis/arthritis-diet/anti-inflammatory/gluten-free-diet.php
- http://www.huffingtonpost.com/amy-myers-md-/effects-of-gluten-on-the-body_b_3672275.html

GMO FOODS

- Natural Solutions Magazine, article by Mike Snow, October, 2015
- http://www.takepart.com/article/2015/11/25/gmo-salmon-costco
- http://www.nongmoproject.org/learn-more/

INFLAMMATION

- Resources: The Anti-Inflammation Zone, Dr. Barry Sears, pg 12, 22; Systematic review and meta-analysis of clinical trials of the effects of low carbohydrate diets on cardiovascular risk factors; A low-carbohydrate, ketogenic diet versus a low-fat diet to treat obesity and hyper-lipidemia: a randomized, controlled trial; Very-low-carbohydrate ketogenic diet v. low-fat diet for long-term weight loss: a meta-analysis of randomized controlled trials

- https://chriskresser.com/how-inflammation-makes-you-fat-and-diabetic-and-vice-versa/
- http://www.marksdailyapple.com/what-is-inflammation/#axzz47KITSRDL

LEGUMES (BEANS / SOY / PEANUTS)

- http://wellnessmama.com/2029/are-beans-healthy/
- http://drclydewilson.typepad.com/drclydewilson/2011/02/paleo-diet-is-incompetent-legumes-are-not-anti-nutrients.html
- Peanuts: http://kimberlysnyder.com/blog/2012/10/25/peanuts-health-food-or-hazardous-to-your-health/
- Peanuts: (Good and Bad) http://articles.mercola.com/sites/articles/archive/2003/08/20/peanuts-health.aspx
- http://www.drweil.com/drw/u/QAA401607/Whats-Wrong-With-Peanut-Skin.html
- http://chriskresser.com/are-legumes-paleo/
- http://www.drweil.com/drw/u/ART03206/Cooking-With-Legumes.html
- http://www.mayoclinic.org/healthy-lifestyle/nutrition-and-healthy-eating/in-depth/legumes/art-20044278?pg=2

MEATS

- http://www.eatwild.com/basics.html (Understanding Grass-Fed, pastured. Resources for purchasing)
- http://www.neysbigsky.com (Grass-fed and organic meats, shipped to you)
- http://grasslandbeef.com (Grass-fed and organic meats, shipped to you)

MSG AND OTHER ADDITIVES

- http://www.mayoclinic.org/healthy-lifestyle/nutrition-and-healthy-eating/expert-answers/monosodium-glutamate/faq-20058196
- http://www.foodrenegade.com/msg-dangerous-science/
- Food dye: http://articles.mercola.com/sites/articles/archive/2011/02/24/are-you-or-your-family-eating-toxic-food-dyes.aspx
- http://www.doctoroz.com/article/food-dyes-are-they-safe
- Additives to avoid: http://foodmatters.tv/articles-1/top-10-food-additives-to-avoid

NATURAL HEALTH CARE, BEAUTY, AND PERSONAL HYGIENE PRODUCTS

- <u>Natural Solutions</u> Magazine
- https://www.piperwai.com (deodorant – it really WORKS!!)

- www.youngliving.com (essential oils)
- www.ewg.org/skindeep/ (choosing products that are safe)
- www.ombotanical.com (organic, non-toxic skin care)
- www.juicebeauty.com (organic, non-toxic skin care and cosmetics)
- www.earthsbeauty.com (organic, non-toxic skin care and cosmetics)
- www.suzannesomers.com (organic, non-toxic skin care and cosmetics)
- www.100percentpure.com(organic, non-toxic skin care and cosmetics)
- www.purpleprairie.com (natural skin are, bug sprays, sunscreen)

NON-TOXIC CLEANING AND LAUNDRY

- http://www.ewg.org/guides/cleaners
- http://www.wholefoodsmarket.com/about-our-products/premium-body-care-standards
- http://eartheasy.com/live_nontoxic_solutions.htm (making your own)
- http://www.keeperofthehome.org/2013/06/homemade-all-natural-cleaning-recipes.html (making your own)
- Young Living – www.youngliving.com
- Seventh Generation Products
- The Honest Company
- J.R. Watkins
- Meyers Clean Day
- Earth Friendly
- Planet
- Simple Green

NUTS

- http://articles.mercola.com/sites/articles/archive/2012/03/29/raw-nuts-health-benefits.aspx
- http://www.wisebread.com/the-best-and-worst-nuts-by-nutrition-and-price

OILS

- Which to cook with: http://chriskresser.com/5-fats-you-should-be-cooking-with-but-may-not-be/
- Healthy cooking oils: https://authoritynutrition.com/healthy-cooking-oils/
- Healthy cooking oils: http://foodmatters.tv/articles-1/whats-the-best-oil-to-cook-with
- Canola Oil: http://articles.mercola.com/herbal-oils/canola-oil.aspx
- Olive Oil: https://authoritynutrition.com/extra-virgin-olive-oil/
- Coconut Oil: https://authoritynutrition.com/why-is-coconut-oil-good-for-you/

- Avocado Oil: http://www.today.com/food/avocado-oil-new-coconut-oil-how-do-you-use-it-t65581

ORGANIC EATING

- http://www.organic.org
- http://www.ewg.org/foodnews/list/
- http://www.toxicsaction.org/problems-and-solutions/pesticides
- http://foodrevolution.org/blog/is-organic-better/
- http://strongertogether.coop/fresh-from-the-source/farming-and-production/four-reasons-that-organic-food-is-better-than-conventional/
- http://www.mayoclinic.org/healthy-lifestyle/nutrition-and-healthy-eating/in-depth/organic-food/art-20043880
- http://www.prevention.com/food/healthy-eating-tips/top-reasons-choose-organic-foods
- Soil: http://www.scientificamerican.com/article/soil-depletion-and-nutrition-loss/
- Pesticides: https://www.geneticliteracyproject.org/2015/12/07/myth-busting-on-pesticides-despite-demonization-organic-farmers-widely-use-them

ORGANIC, PURE SPICES

- http://www.spicely.com
- Whole Foods
- Thrive Market

PLASTIC

- http://articles.mercola.com/sites/articles/archive/2011/11/16/practical-options-to-store-your-food-without-contaminating-them-with-plastics.aspx
- http://www.webmd.com/food-recipes/cookware-plastics-shoppers-guide-to-food-safety
- http://science.time.com/2011/03/08/study-even-bpa-free-plastics-leach-endocrine-disrupting-chemicals/

PROBIOTICS

- The Road to Perfect Health, by Brenda Watson
- http://probioticamerica.com
- http://probiotics.mercola.com/probiotics.html
- http://florastor.com/about/

- http://www.renewlife.com/ultimate-flora-probiotics.html?gclid=Cj0KEQjwr5G5BRD_n-T0pf7x4ucBEiQAlxHOP_vbBFWYmvmXPC6p23SkFu94r9f9OeEgbmEz3UycHdMaAmH-s8P8HAQ
- Leaky Gut: http://draxe.com/4-steps-to-heal-leaky-gut-and-autoimmune-disease/
- Immune system in gut: http://ecowatch.com/2015/02/26/gut-health-boost-immune-system/

SEAFOOD BUYING AND INFORMATION

- http://www.seafoodwatch.org
- http://www.montereybayaquarium.org/cr/seafoodwatch.aspx
- http://www.seafoodwatch.org/seafood-recommendations/our-app

SHOPPING: SOURCES FOR ON-LINE, HEALTHY AND ORGANIC FOOD PRODUCTS

- https://thrivemarket.com/giftbox/cocohome
- http://www.vitacost.com/vitacostbrandcategories/?csrc=SITEREF-linkshare
- http://www.sunfood.com
- http://www.amazon.com/Natural-Organic-Grocery/b?node=51537011

SOY

- https://authoritynutrition.com/is-soy-bad-for-you-or-good/
- http://www.foodrenegade.com/dangers-of-soy/
- https://www.mercola.com/article/soy/avoid_soy.htm
- http://www.thehealthyhomeeconomist.com/170-scientific-reasons-to-lose-the-soy-in-your-diet/
- http://thewholejourney.com/soy-the-good-the-bad-and-the-ugly
- http://www.veganhealth.org/articles/soy_wth
- http://www.livestrong.com/article/352117-amino-acids-in-soy-protein/

SUGAR

- <u>Sugar Shock</u>, Connie Bennett, C.H.H.C., with Stephen Sinatra, M.D.
- http://mobile.nytimes.com/2016/09/13/well/eat/how-the-sugar-industry-shifted-blame-to-fat.html?_r=1&referer=
- http://drhyman.com/blog/2014/03/06/top-10-big-ideas-detox-sugar/
- http://wellnessmama.com/15/harmful-effects-of-sugar/
- http://articles.mercola.com/sugar-side-effects.aspx

- http://www.foxnews.com/health/2016/01/06/study-links-sugar-to-cancer-how-to-reduce-your-risk.html
- http://www.totalhealthmagazine.com/Diet-and-Nutrition/Sugar-Is-Pro-Inflammatory.html
- http://www.healthline.com/health/food-nutrition/experts-is-sugar-addictive-drug
- http://ajcn.nutrition.org/content/82/3/675
- Stevia: Brands that are pure: http://food.allwomenstalk.com/brands-of-stevia-that-are-the-best-tasting-and-the-best-for-you

VITAMINS AND NUTRIENTS

- Designs for Health http://www.designsforhealth.com
- Life Extension www.lef.org
- http://www.mercola.com
- https://www.gardenoflife.com/content/
- Antioxidant/Vit C: http://foodmatters.tv/product/superfood-vitamin-c
- http://www.integrativepro.com
- http://www.prlabs.com
- Fiber http://www.helpforibs.com/shop/suplmts/acacia.asp
- http://articles.mercola.com/sites/articles/archive/2014/01/20/food-nutrients-vitamin-supplements.aspx
- http://articles.mercola.com/antioxidants.aspx

WATER

- http://www.rd.com/health/diet-weight-loss/rethink-what-you-drink/
- http://www.mercola.com/article/water.htm
- http://www.allaboutwater.org/filtered-water.html
- Infused water: http://wellnessmama.com/3607/herb-fruit-infused-water/
- http://greatist.com/health/health-benefits-water

WEBSITES ON NUTRITION, HEALTHY LIVING, RECIPES

- www.exercisecoach.com
- www.foodmatters.com
- www.cleaneating.com
- www.elanaspantry.com
- www.mercola.com
- www.jonnybowden.com
- www.drhyman.com

- http://www.anh-usa.org
- http://meljoulwan.com/2010/02/14/dino-chowpaleo-recipe-roundup/
- http://simplynourishedrecipes.com
- http://www.thewholesmiths.com
- http://www.godairyfree.org
- https://thrivemarket.com/giftbox/cocohome
- nomnompaleo.com
- wholelifeeating.com
- http://www.rubiesandradishes.com
- http://www.thewholesmiths.com
- http://www.godairyfree.org
- http://deliciouslyorganic.net
- http://www.100daysofrealfood.com

About the Author

After suffering from chronic digestive issues for years, Gerianne Cygan devoted herself to researching nutrition and health. In 2000, she and her husband, Brian, cofounded the Exercise Coach to share their life-changing fitness principles with others.

Cygan has extensively studied major diet theories, and in 2014 she received the title of Certified Health Coach from the Institute of Integrative Nutrition.

Cygan enjoys cooking and spending time with her husband and three children.

Made in the USA
Middletown, DE
18 July 2019